D1709129

Tai Chi Chuan

....

Medicine and Sport Science

Vol. 52

Tai Chi Chuan

State of the Art in International Research

Volume Editor

Youlian Hong, Hong Kong

38 figures, and 26 tables, 2008

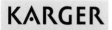

Basel · Freiburg · Paris · London · New York ·
Bangalore · Bangkok · Singapore · Tokyo · Sydney

Medicine and Sport Science

Founder and Editor from 1969 to 1984: E. Jokl†, Lexington, Ky.

••••••••••••••••••••••

Prof. Youlian Hong

Department of Sports Science and Physical Education
The Chinese University of Hong Kong
Shatin, Hong Kong (China)

Library of Congress Cataloging-in-Publication Data

Tai chi chuan : state of the art in international research / volume editor,
Youlian Hong.
     p. ; cm. – (Medicine and sport science, ISSN 0254-5020 ; v. 52)
   Includes bibliographical references and indexes.
   ISBN 978-3-8055-8489-0 (hard cover : alk. paper)
   1. Tai chi–Health aspects. I. Hong, Youlian, 1946– II. Series.
   [DNLM: 1. Tai Ji. 2. Exercise Therapy–methods. W1 ME649Q v.52 2008 /
WB 541 T129 2008]
   RA781.85.T35 2008
   613.7′148–dc22

                                                2008004151

Bibliographic Indices. This publication is listed in bibliographic services, including Current Contents® and Index Medicus.

© Copyright 2008 by S. Karger AG, P.O. Box, CH–4009 Basel (Switzerland)
www.karger.com
Printed in Switzerland on acid-free and non-aging paper (ISO 9706) by Reinhardt Druck, Basel
ISSN 0254–5020
ISBN 978–3–8055–8489–0

....

Contents

Contents

Preface

Tai Chi Chuan (TCC, TC, T'ai Chi, or Taiji) was originally developed as a form of martial arts. It has been used for centuries in China as a health exercise for a wide age range but has particularly been popular among the elderly. The basic exercise involved in TCC is a series of individual movements that are linked together in a continuous manner and that flow smoothly from one movement to another. Deep breathing and mental concentration are also required to achieve harmony between the body and the mind in TCC. Thus, TCC is not only a physical activity, but it also involves the training of the nervous system. In particular, people practice TCC for the development of mind-body interaction, breath regulation with body movement, eye-hand coordination, and a peaceful state of mind. In addition, TCC can be practiced any time and in any place because it needs neither wide space nor any equipment. The simple, soft, and fluid movements of TCC are ideal for older people regardless of previous exercise experience. Today, it has spread to many countries worldwide, and millions of people in both Eastern and Western countries and cultures are practicing TCC. More importantly, it has been widely accepted as an exercise form for health and fitness benefits.

To our knowledge, the first paper in English that presented an experimental study on TCC was published in the 1980s. With the prevalence of an aging population worldwide and with the concomitant increases in expenditure for the relief of chronic disease and disability, interest in TCC has continued to grow. Published results from well-controlled studies about the effects of TCC, particularly those focusing on the elderly, have added to an understanding of the characteristics of TCC movement and its impact on health. Based on the published literature, TCC can seemingly equal all of the exercise demands that elderly people require. Additionally, TCC seems to have the potential to considerably reduce expenditure associated with poor health because it facilitates a lifestyle that promotes the well-being of people of all ages. However, before endorsing these broad observations, two relevant questions must be addressed. What evidence actually exists to suggest that TCC affords any health benefits? Then, if such benefits indeed exist, what are their underlying mechanisms? In light of these, the aim of this book is to reflect current studies focusing on the characteristics of this intriguing form of exercise, their impact on the participants' health, and the scientific basis of the beneficial effects of TCC on health and fitness.

This book is the first collection of scientific studies on TCC in the world. It is organized into four sections, each containing four to seven chapters, totaling to twenty-two chapters. The first section addresses 'the biomechanical and physiological characteristics of Tai Chi' in seven chapters. The opening chapter highlights the temporal characteristics of foot movement in TCC by Youlian Hong and colleagues, which is followed by the chapter exploring heart rate responses and oxygen consumption during TCC practice by Ching Lan and colleagues. The third chapter, by Dong Qing Xu and colleagues, introduces TCC and muscle strength and endurance in older people. Then Ge Wu discusses the muscle action patterns and isokinetic knee extensor strength of older TCC practitioners. The fifth chapter, contributed by Ruth Taylor-Piliae and colleagues, describes how TCC aids in improving aerobic capacity, while in the sixth chapter, Everard W. Thornton discusses on how TCC helps in improving cardiorespiratory capacity. The section concludes with the chapter that describes the effects of a traditional taiji/qigong curriculum on older adults' immune response to influenza vaccine as contributed by Yang Yang and colleagues.

The second section highlights the benefits of TCC in terms of balance control and fall prevention in five chapters. The section begins with the chapter on TCC and proprioceptive behavior in older people as contributed by Jing Xian Li and colleagues. The second chapter, written by Strawberry Gatts, addresses the issue of neural mechanism underlying balance control in TCC. Then William W.N. Tsang and Christina W.Y. Hui-Chan discuss how repeated practice of Tai Chi can improve limb joint proprioception, integration of neural signals in the central nervous system for balance control, and motor output at the level of knee muscles. The fourth chapter, contributed by Alice M.K. Wong and Ching Lan, discusses the effects of TCC on balance and posture control in elderly people. Finally, Peter A. Harmer and Fuzhong Li describe TCC and fall prevention in older people.

The third section focuses on the mental health and social aspects of TCC and consists of four chapters. Yong 'Tai' Wang addresses TCC and the improvement of mental and physical health among college students, which is followed by the chapter on the effects of TCC on depressive symptoms in elderly people by Kee-Lee Chou. In the third chapter, Matthew Kwai-sang Yau discusses TCC and the improvement of health and wellbeing in older adults. The section ends with the chapter written by Robert B. Wall who focuses on teaching TCC with mindfulness-based stress reduction to middle school children in the inner city, which is a review of related literature and approaches.

Six chapters in the fourth or the last section demonstrate the application of TCC in clinical intervention. For this purpose, Penelope J. Klein introduces TCC in the management of Parkinson's disease and Alzheimer's disease, and Ching Lan and colleagues address TCC training for individuals with coronary heart disease. Then, Gloria Y. Yeh and colleagues describe TCC in individuals with chronic heart failure, and Karen M. Mustian and colleagues show the effects of TCC on functional capacity and quality of life among breast cancer survivors. The fifth chapter, contributed by Chenchen Wang, is focused on the topic 'Tai Chi Improves Pain and Functional Status in Adults with Rheumatoid Arthritis: Results of a Pilot Single-Blinded Randomized Controlled Trial'. Finally, the book ends with the chapter on the effects of TCC on diabetic individuals as reported by Jing Hao Wang.

The contributors to this book are recognized scholars who have all provided original and relevant research articles to the international TCC literature. The chapters they contributed not only provide good examples of how to use TCC in health promotion but also explore the underlying mechanism of the beneficial effects of TCC. The editor is indebted to them for their high-quality contributions.

Youlian Hong

Hong Y (ed): Tai Chi Chuan. State of the Art in International Research.
Med Sport Sci. Basel, Karger, 2008, vol 52, pp 1–11

·······················

Temporal Characteristics of Foot Movement in Tai Chi Exercise

Youlian Hong[a], *De Wei Mao*[a,b], *Jing Xian Li*[a,c]

[a]Department of Sports Science and Physical Education, The Chinese University of
Hong Kong, Hong Kong; [b]Shandong Institute of Physical Education and Sports, Jinan,
China; [c]School of Human Kinetics, University of Ottawa, Ottawa, Canada

---

Abstract

The concept of proper foot movement is always emphasized in the practice of Tai Chi.
Sixteen experienced Tai Chi practitioners participated in this study. Each subject practiced
the whole set of 42-form Tai Chi movements and the performance was video-recorded and
analyzed. The study found that Tai Chi is performed with the interchange of seven support
patterns and six step directions of the foot. Compared with normal walking, there is a bigger
percentage of time spent performing double support and less percentage of time spent performing single support movements in Tai Chi. However, the average duration of each support
movement is longer and the change from one type of support to another is slower. In Tai Chi,
the duration of steps in each direction is short and there are frequent changes from one direction to another. Tai Chi was found to be more effective than walking in simulating the gait
challenges that are encountered in daily activities.

Copyright © 2008 S. Karger AG, Basel

Tai Chi is a Chinese form of exercise that is derived from martial arts folk
traditions. It entails extended and natural postures, slow and even motions, light
and steady movements, and curved, flowing lines of performance. Several studies have shown the beneficial effects of Tai Chi exercise on muscle strength,
flexibility, balance control, and prevention of falls [1–3]. According to the theory of Tai Chi, foot posture and movement are the foundation of the whole-
body posture, and the concept of proper position and direction is always
emphasized [4]. Studies on kinematics of Tai Chi have focused mainly on single
movements [5–7]. Little is known about the kinematics of the whole set of Tai
Chi movements, especially on the foot movement characteristics.

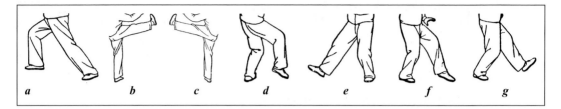

Fig. 1. Foot support patterns: full double-limb support (***a***), single-limb left support (***b***), single-limb right support (***c***), left support with right toe touch (***d***), left support with right heel touch (***e***), right support with left toe touch (***f***), and right support with left heel touch (***g***).

Walking is the basic form of ambulation in daily activities. Several studies have demonstrated the positive effects of walking training programs on postural stability [8], muscle strength [9], and cardiorespiratory responses [10] in elderly people. Regular walking for elderly people has been recommended for increasing physical activity and decreasing the risk for falls [11]. The purposes of this study were to compare Tai Chi with normal walking in terms of temporal parameters of support pattern and step direction of foot. It is hoped that such comparison would enhance our understanding why Tai Chi exercise has beneficial effects on balance and muscle strength. The 42-form Tai Chi was selected for study because all of the basic and typical movements from various Tai Chi schools are combined in this form, which is used in national and international competitions.

Method

Subjects

Sixteen gender-matched, experienced Tai Chi practitioners (8 female and 8 male, age 23.07 ± 5.53 years, body height 166.0 ± 7.6 cm, body weight 62.27 ± 7.87 kg, experience 8.09 ± 5.72 years) with no previous diseases or injuries 1 year before the study were recruited. All subjects completed consent forms before testing.

Procedure

The subjects were asked to perform the whole set of 42-form Tai Chi once at a self-selected training pace and walk a 15-meter pathway in three trials at a normal self-selected speed. Two digital video cameras (JVC 9800) with 50-Hz frequency were synchronized to record the subject's movements during the whole set of Tai Chi performance, with one camera (A) focusing on the lower extremities and the other (B) on the whole body. Before testing, the subjects were given ample time to warm up.

In accordance with the traditional description of foot movement in Tai Chi [4], the foot support pattern was divided into seven categories (fig. 1). These categories are: (1) full

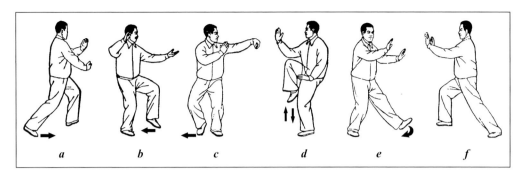

Fig. 2. Categories of step direction: stepping forward – an anterior movement of one foot in relation to the support foot (***a***), stepping backward – a posterior movement of one foot in relation to the support foot (***b***), stepping sideways – a lateral movement of one foot in relation to the support foot (***c***), up and down stepping – upward lifting of one foot above the knee height of the support leg (***d***), stepping turning – pivotal rotation (medial or lateral) on the support foot with stepping action of other foot (***e***), and stepping fixing or fixed step – both feet are fixed to the ground with no foot movement (***f***).

double-limb support, (2) left single-limb support, (3) right single-limb support, (4) left support with right toe touch, (5) left support with right heel touch, (6) right support with left toe touch, and (7) right support with left heel touch.

Likewise, the stepping direction of foot was divided into six categories (fig. 2). These categories were: (1) stepping forward – an anterior movement of one foot in relation to the stance foot, (2) stepping backward – a posterior movement of one foot in relation to the stance foot, (3) stepping sideways – a lateral movement of one foot in relation to the stance foot, (4) up and down stepping – upward lifting of one foot above the knee height of the stance leg, (5) stepping turning – pivotal rotation (medial or lateral) on one stance foot followed by stepping action of the other foot, and (6) stepping fixing, or fixed step – both feet are fixed to the ground with no foot movement.

The APAS motion analysis system (Ariel Dynamics Inc., Trabuco Canyon, Calif., USA) was used to analyze the videotapes frame by frame. The videotape from camera A was used to determine the time components of foot movement in relation to the ground while the videotape from camera B was used to identify which Tai Chi movement was performed. To establish high reliability, three principles were followed to determine each support pattern and step direction: (1) the two video views principle – two captured video images were played in separate windows on the same screen, and each view was confirmed before determining the frames that recorded the beginning and end of each support pattern or step direction; (2) the whole-body principle – because Tai Chi movement is the coordination of all parts of the body, the motion of each body segment was considered, and (3) the continuous movement principle – the previous and next movements were considered when determining the present movement because the Tai Chi movement is even and continuous.

Table 1. Intraclass correlation coefficients for the foot movement characteristics during the 42-form TC exercise

Foot movement characteristics	Total duration	Duration of single foot movement
Support pattern	0.93	0.92
Step direction	0.85	0.83

Data Analysis

In Tai Chi, three dependent variables were determined. They are as follows: (1) 'Total duration' of each support pattern and step direction, which was the sum of all movement durations of respective support patterns and step directions in the whole set of Tai Chi. (2) 'Percentage duration' of movements of each support pattern and step direction, which was the 'total duration' of respective support patterns and step directions divided by the time spent performing the whole set of Tai Chi. (3) 'Average duration' of movements of each support pattern and step direction, which was the 'total duration' of respective support patterns and step directions divided by the number of repetition of this movement in the whole set of Tai Chi.

In normal walking, the movements are cyclic, and a complete gait cycle contains two double-limb support and two (left and right) single-limb support movements. Due to the quasi-symmetric movements of the left and right body limbs in the normal gait cycle, the two double support movements were combined. This leads to one double limb, one left single-limb, and one right single-limb support pattern to be considered in studying the temporal parameters of normal walking. The following two dependent variables were determined: (1) 'Average duration' of each support pattern, which was the duration of movements of respective support patterns in the 'average gait cycle'. In this study, for each walk trial, three complete gait cycles were selected and averaged to represent respective walk trials. The average gait cycles of the three walk trials were then further averaged to yield the 'average gait cycle' mentioned above. (2) 'Percentage duration' of movements of each support pattern, which was the 'average duration' of respective support patterns divided by the time spent performing the 'average gait cycle'.

Because these variables are continuous measurements throughout the whole set of Tai Chi movements using videotapes, intraclass correlation coefficients (ICC(3,k)) were calculated [12] to determine the reliability of data obtained in the study. An independent t test was used to detect any differences between males and females and between Tai Chi and normal walking in each of the dependent variables. SPSS for Windows software was used, and the significance level was set at 0.05.

Results

Based on the results obtained by the two researchers, statistical analysis showed that all of the ICCs were greater than 0.80 (table 1), which indicated that the measurement reliability was high. After this process, the data obtained by the two researchers were averaged.

Table 2. Duration variables of support patterns in the 42-form TC exercise

Support pattern	Total duration, s		Percentage duration		Average duration, s	
	mean	SD	mean	SD	mean	SD
Full double-limb support	115.62	23.76	33.63	4.91	1.86	0.30
Left single-limb support	60.63	9.85	17.90	1.55	1.94	0.31
Right single-limb right support	60.43	9.99	17.83	2.09	1.95	0.31
Left support with right toe touch	22.58	3.66	6.68	0.99	0.55	0.06
Left support with right heel touch	25.60	4.85	7.61	1.30	0.90	0.13
Right support with left toe touch	24.97	4.10	7.36	1.00	0.59	0.09
Right support with left heel touch	30.42	6.21	8.99	1.59	0.95	0.10

Table 3. Direction variables of step movements in the 42-form TC exercise

Step direction	Total duration, s		Percentage duration, %		Average duration, s	
	mean	SD	mean	SD	mean	SD
Forward	67.78	15.43	19.99	3.18	2.10	0.73
Backward	16.07	6.70	4.84	1.83	1.95	0.84
Sideways	53.72	24.34	13.94	7.11	2.08	0.99
Up and down	43.97	10.61	13.53	2.26	4.38	1.02
Turning	66.42	25.03	17.57	3.80	0.97	0.33
Fixing	92.47	31.94	30.11	6.91	1.77	0.90

The independent T test demonstrated that there was no significant difference between male and female subjects on each of the dependent variables. All of the parameters of the male and female subjects were pooled and averaged for further analysis. The support pattern and step direction-related variables in the 42-form Tai Chi performance are shown in table 2 and table 3, respectively. The support pattern-related variables of normal walking are shown in table 4.

During the practice of Tai Chi, the percentage duration of all double-limb supports was 64.26 (6.96)%, which was the sum of durations of all full double-limb supports, all left supports with other toe touch, all left supports with other heel touch, all right supports with other toe touch, and all right supports with other heel touch. The average duration of double-limb support movement of all categories was 0.97 (0.14) s. As mentioned above, it is useful to compare the

Table 4. Duration variables of support patterns in the gait cycle of normal walking

Support pattern	Average duration, s		Percentage duration	
	mean	SD	mean	SD
Double-limb support	0.26	0.20	23.22	3.21
Left single-limb support	0.42	0.14	38.27	2.45
Right single-limb support	0.42	0.17	38.50	2.37

unique foot movement characteristics of Tai Chi with normal walking. The independent t test shows that there is significant difference in percentage duration of movements of each support pattern between the whole set of 42-form Tai Chi and normal walking ($p < 0.01$; fig. 3). Meanwhile, there is significant difference in the average duration of movements of each support pattern in the whole set of 42-form Tai Chi and the average gait cycle ($p < 0.01$; fig. 4). The duration of average gait cycle was 1.10 (0.11) s.

Discussion

Supporting Pattern

Figure 3 demonstrates that the set of 42-form Tai Chi has longer percentage duration in double-limb support patterns (64.26 vs. 23.220%) and shorter percentage duration in single-limb support patterns (17.87 vs. 38.39%) than normal walking. The purposes of walking are to transport the body safely and efficiently across the ground using both legs and to provide both support and propulsion [13], whereas Tai Chi practice emphasizes stable, balanced, slow, and even motions [4]. More time spent performing double-limb support may be beneficial to maintain a balanced and even movement.

Some studies have demonstrated that Tai Chi exercise improves balance performance by increasing balance time [14, 15] and reducing the mean sway displacement of the center of pressure [16, 17] during single-limb support tests. This improved balance performance occurs because standing on one leg is a common posture in the practice of Tai Chi [17]. Our study showed that the durations of left single-limb (1.94 s) and right single-limb (1.95 s) support were the two largest values among the support patterns (table 2) and were much longer than in normal walking (0.42 s; fig. 4). These results also supported the report

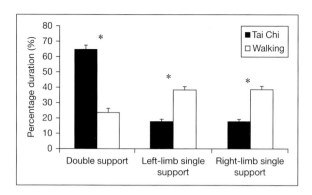

Fig. 3. Comparison of percentage duration of movements of each support pattern between the whole set of 42-form Tai Chi and normal walking. Asterisk denotes significant difference between Tai Chi and normal walking. *$p < 0.01$.

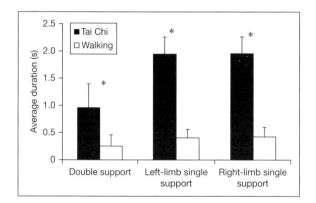

Fig. 4. Comparison of average duration of movements of each support pattern between the whole set of 42-form Tai Chi and normal walking. Asterisk denotes significant difference between Tai Chi and normal walking. *$p < 0.01$.

of [6], who found that there was a longer duration of single-limb stance time in the defined 'Tai Chi gait' than in normal walking. In this connection, the longer time spent performing each single-limb support may contribute to the improved single-limb stance balance ability.

As shown in table 2, the average duration of each of the 5 double-limb support patterns in Tai Chi (1.86, 0.55, 0.90, 0.59, and 0.95 s) was longer than the average duration of each double-limb support in normal walking (0.13 s; table 4).

These data revealed that in addition to single-limb support, various double support patterns have also longer duration than in normal walking. The increased
period in each support pattern reduced the speed of motion and slowed the
changes from one pattern to another, thus prolonging the duration of contraction
of the relative muscles, which may improve the strength and endurance of those
muscles [5, 7]. In addition, the performance of Tai Chi relies on full double-limb
weight bearing, full single-limb weight bearing, and single-limb weight bearing
with other toe or heel semi-weight-bearing maneuvers. These patterns demand a
high balance control capacity. The balance control of the center of gravity and the
accurate adjustment of foot position during the practice of Tai Chi forces more
muscles to be involved in the exercise, which may lead to increased muscle
strength [6, 7].

Stepping Pattern
Stepping backward is used in everyday activities such as approaching a sitting position in a chair. Some researchers have reported that backward walking
has modified speed, and stride length [13, 18], increasing electromyography
magnitude and patterns [13], and increased cardiorespiratory and metabolic
responses [19] when compared with forward walking. Thus, it has been suggested that backward walking should be considered as a rehabilitation tool to
improve daily functional abilities [18, 19]. Tai Chi exercise includes backward
walking that may improve muscle strength and enhance the backward stepping
ability that is needed in daily activities.
Lateral instability has induced a sizable proportion of falls to the side,
which are most likely to result in hip fracture injuries [20]. One of the strategies
to compensate for the destabilization in the mediolateral direction is side-
stepping [21]. With increasing age, older adults consistently take more steps to
recover equilibrium than younger adults [22]. Elderly people tend to use additional limb-movement reactions after the initial stepping reaction. That is, the
new base of support established by the initial stepping reaction is insufficient to
capture and arrest the motion of the center of mass [22]. During Tai Chi exercise, the sideways movement with the coordination of trunk and upper limbs
may match the demand of stepping sideways when perturbations occur.
Obstacles can be found indoors or outdoors, in flooring or sidewalk
paving, at carpet edges, or in the form of electrical cords or door thresholds
[23]. It has been shown that almost 50% of falls in community-dwelling older
adults occur during destabilizing activities such as stepping over an obstacle or
negotiating a raised surface [24]. Elderly people will be challenged by these
destabilizing activities, which had a typical single-limb support pattern movement, because these activities require considerable demands on the musculoskeletal system and thus pose a greater threat to stability. Chen et al. [23]

reported that the foot clearance over an obstacle is approximately 3 times greater than in level gait. Older adults exhibited a significantly more conservative strategy when crossing obstacles, with slower crossing speed, shorter step length, and shorter obstacle-heel-strike distance. In contrast, the stepping up and down movement, in which one foot is supported with the other foot raised from the ground above knee level and then downward to the ground, is one of the movements in Tai Chi exercise. Practicing Tai Chi may help elderly people to manage with those challenging activities such as stepping over an obstacle and negotiating a raised surface because they have already simulated and practiced similar movements in Tai Chi exercise.

Turning is a powerful indicator of falling and is a characteristic that changes with age [25]. Cumming and Klineberg [26] examined the association between a history of falls and the risk for hip fracture in 412 older adults and identified the characteristics of falls that are related to hip fracture. They found that people who fell while performing a standing turn test were 7.9 times more likely than those who did not fall to have a subsequent fall resulting in a hip fracture. Thigpen et al. [25] studied movement characteristics during turning and found that elderly people took more steps and more time than young people to accomplish a turn. There was an almost total absence of a pivot type of turn in the elderly group. In the practice of Tai Chi, the turning maneuvers include one-foot support with other toe touching and internal or external pivoting, one-foot support with the other heel touching and internal or external pivoting, and even each foot touching with internal or external pivoting simultaneously. All kinds of pivoting maneuvers and many turning movements involved in Tai Chi are likely to improve the ability of turning.

Our results showed that the durations of stepping forward, backward, sideways, up and down, turning, and fixing were 2.10, 1.95, 2.08, 4.38, 0.97, and 1.77 s, respectively (table 3). These results revealed that the duration of each stepping direction was just a few seconds, which allows the directions of stepping to be adjusted frequently. The challenges of maintaining balance during daily life are often likely to demand changes in the base of support to enhance stability. Successful balance recovery by means of stepping requires accurate control of the foot movement as well as controlling the motion of the center of mass to arrest it within the boundaries of the new base of support established by the step [27]. Thus, compensatory stepping in all directions is an important strategy for preserving stability [28]. The Tai Chi movements in our study were combinations of stepping forward, backward, sideways, up and down, turning, and fixing that are similar to challenges to balance control that are encountered in daily activities. To prevent falls among elderly people, Campbell et al. [29] developed a home-based exercise program that included walking backward and sideways, turning around, and stepping over an object. They found that the program improved physical function and was effective in reducing falls and injuries in elderly people.

Tai Chi is characterized by slow and even 3-dimensional motions and involves the coordination of all parts of the body [4]. In our study, only isolated foot movements were selected, with no consideration of trunk or upper extremity movements, which provided limited information on the kinematics of Tai Chi movements.

Conclusions

Temporal characteristics of seven support patterns and six step directions of foot during Tai Chi exercise were determined. In Tai Chi exercise, all double- and single-limb support movements were performed slower as compared with normal walking, and there was a slow change from one support pattern to another. The duration of step in each direction was short and there was a frequent change of step from one direction to another. Various support patterns changing slowly, combined with various step directions changing fully, may be more effective than walking at simulating the gait challenges that are encountered during daily activities.

Acknowledgements

The work described in this paper was fully supported by a grant from the Research Grants Council of the Hong Kong Special Administrative Region (project CUHK4360/00H).

References

1   Hong YL, Li JX, Robinson: Balance control, flexibility, and cardiorespiratory fitness among older Tai Chi practitioners. Br J Sports Med 2000;34:29–34.
2   Li F, Harmer P, Fisher KJ, McAuley E, Chaumeton N, Eckstrom E, Wilson NL: Tai Chi and fall reduction in oldewr adults: a randomized controlled trial. J Gerontol A Biol Sci Med Sci 2005;60: 187–194.
3   Tsang WW, Hui-Chan CW: Comparison of muscle torque, balance, and confidence in older tai chi and healthy adults. Med Sci Sports Exerc 2005;37:280–289.
4   People's Sports Publishing: Tai Chi Chuan Exercise. Beijing, China: People's Sports Publishing, 2000.
5   Chan SP, Luk TC, Hong YL: Kinematic and electromyographic analysis of the push movement in Tai Chi. Br J Sports Med 2003;37:339–344.
6   Wu G, Liu W, Hitt J, Millon D: Spatial, temporal and muscle action patterns of Tai Chi gait. J Electromyogr Kinesiol 2004;14:343–354.
7   Xu DQ, Li JX, Hong YL: Tai Chi movement and proprioceptive training: a kinematics and EMG analysis. Res Sports Med 2003;11:129–143.
8   Melzer I, Benjuya N, Kaplanski J: Effects of regular walking on postural stability in the elderly. Gerontology 2003;49:240–245.

9   Carmeli E, Kessel S, Coleman R, Ayalon M: Effects of a treadmill walking program on muscle strength and balance in elderly people with Down syndrome. J Gerontol A Biol Sci Med Sci 2002;57:M106–M110.

10 Shin Y: The effects of a walking exercise program on physical function and emotional state of elderly Korean women. Public Health Nurs 1999;16:146–154.

11 Cooper KM, Bilbrew D, Dubbert PM, et al: Health barriers to walking for exercise in elderly primary care. Geriatr Nurs 2001;22:258–262.

12 Dite W, Temple VA: Development of a clinical measure of turning for older adults. Am J Phys Med Rehabil 2002;81:857–866.

13 Winter DA: The Biomechanical and Motor Control of Human Gait. Waterloo, Canada: University of Waterloo Press, 1991.

14 Schaller KJ: Tai Chi Chih: an exercise option for older adults. J Gerontol Nurs 1996;22:12–17.

15 Tse AK, Bailey DM: Tai Chi and postural control in the well elderly. Am J Occup Ther 1991;46: 295–300.

16 Judge JO, Lindsey C, Underwood M, et al: Balance improvements in older women: effects of exercise training. Phys Ther 1993;73:254–265.

17 Margaret KM, Pui LN: Mediolateral sway in single-leg stance is the best discriminator of balance performance for Tai-Chi practitioners. Arch Phys Med Rehabil 2003;84:683–686.

18 Yocheved L: Age-and gender-related changes in the temporal-spatial characteristics of forwards and backwards gaits. Physiother Res Int 2003;8:131–142.

19 Myatt G, Baxter R, Dougherty R, et al: The cardiopulmonary cost of backward walking at selected speeds. J Orthop Sports Phys Ther 1995;21:132–138.

20 Nevitt MC, Cummings SR: Type of fall and risk of hip and wrist fractures: the study of osteoporotic fractures. J Am Geriatr Soc 1993;41:1226–1234.

21 Maki BE, McIlroy WE: The role of limb movements in maintaining upright stance: the 'change-in-support' strategy. Phys Ther 1997;77:488–507.

22 Maki BE, Edmondstone MA, McIlroy WE: Age-related differences in laterally directed compensatory stepping behavior. J Gerontol A Biol Sci Med Sci 2000;55:M270–M277.

23 Chen HC, Ashton-Miller JA, Alexander NB, Schultz AB: Stepping over obstacles: gait patterns of healthy young and old adults. J Gerontol 1991;46:M196–M203.

24 Lamoureux E, Sparrow WA, Murphy A, Newton RU: The effects of improved strength on obstacle negotiation in community-living older adults. Gait Posture 2003;17:273–283.

25 Thigpen MT, Light KE, Creel GL, Flynn SM: Turning difficulty characteristics of adults aged 65 years or older. Phys Ther 2000;80:1174–1187.

26 Cumming RG, Klineberg RJ: Fall frequency and characteristics and the risk of hip fracture. J Am Geriatr Soc 1994;42:774–778.

27 Maki BE, McIlory WE: The control of foot placement during compensatory stepping reactions: does speed of response take precedence over stability? IEEE Trans Rahabil Eng 1997;7:80–90.

28 McIlroy WE, Maki BE: Age-related changes in compensatory stepping in response to unpredictable perturbations. J Gerontol [A] 1996;51:M289–M296.

29 Campbell AJ, Roberson MC, Gardner MM, et al: Randomised controlled trial of a general practice programme of home based exercise to prevent falls in elderly women. BMJ 1997;315:1065–1069.

Prof. Youlian Hong, PhD
Department of Sports Science, The Chinese University of Hong Kong
Shatin, Hong Kong, SAR (China)
Tel. +1 852 2609 6082, Fax +1 852 2603 5781, E-Mail youlianhong@cuhk.edu.hk

Hong Y (ed): Tai Chi Chuan. State of the Art in International Research.
Med Sport Sci. Basel, Karger, 2008, vol 52, pp 12–19

....

The Exercise Intensity of Tai Chi Chuan

Ching Lan, Ssu-Yuan Chen, Jin-Shin Lai

Department of Physical Medicine and Rehabilitation,
National Taiwan University Hospital and National Taiwan
University, College of Medicine, Taipei, Taiwan

Abstract

Tai Chi Chuan (TC) is a Chinese conditioning exercise and is well-known for its graceful movement. The exercise intensity of TC depends on its training style, posture and duration. Variation in training approaches result in substantial differences in exercise intensity. We have measured heart rate (HR) and oxygen uptake ($\dot{V}O_2$) simultaneously during classical Yang TC practice in 15 male subjects, their heart rate (HR) during TC practice was 58% of the heart rate reserve (HRR), and oxygen uptake ($\dot{V}O_2$) was 55% of the peak oxygen uptake ($\dot{V}O_{2peak}$). The level of blood lactate immediately after TC practice was 3.8 mM, which reflected the level of lactate during TC approximated the onset of blood lactate accumulation (OBLA). In order to evaluate the relative exercise intensity of classical Yang TC, we measured HR responses during TC practice in 100 subjects with age of 25–80 yrs (M/F: 54/46). They were separated into three groups: young (25–44 y/o), middle-aged (45–64 y/o) and elderly (65–80 y/o). During the TC practice, the mean HR of men was 141 ± 12, 132 ± 9 and 120 ± 10 bpm in the young, middle-aged and elderly groups, respectively. Meanwhile, the mean HR of women was 136 ± 10, 126 ± 11 and 115 ± 12 bpm in the young, middle-aged and elderly groups, respectively. Men practiced TC with mean HR corresponding to 57.8 ± 3.7, 56.6 ± 3.4 and $55.1 \pm 3.1\%$ of heart rate reserve (HRR) in the three groups; while that of women corresponding to 52.7 ± 2.8, 51.5 ± 2.6, and $50.3 \pm 2.9\%$ of HRR in the three age groups. The results demonstrate that classical Yang TC is an exercise with moderate intensity, and its exercise intensity is similar across different ages in each gender.

Tai Chi Chuan, a branch of traditional Chinese martial arts, has been widely practiced since the 17th century. During its development, TC gradually evolved into many styles. Among them the Chen style is the oldest, while the

Yang style is the most popular [1]. In recent years, some simplified forms of TC were also developed to shorten the time of learning. Classical TC comprises many complex postures and takes about 30 min to perform a complete set; whereas simplified TC included fewer postures and takes only five minutes to perform. Although simplified TC is easier to learn, it may have lesser training benefits owing to lower exercise intensity and shorter duration.

In the past decade, TC has drawn increased attention owning to its potential health benefits [2–11]. Although TC provides some health benefits, controversy remains because the reported exercise intensity varies in different studies. Some TC training programs only include a few selected postures, and the exercise intensity is much less than a complete set of TC [11, 12]. From the perspective of exercise prescription, the intensity of a 'standard' form of TC should be determined to facilitate its application among different populations. Classical Yang TC is suitable to set as a standard form of TC because it is the original style of Yang TC, developed by Yang Luchan (the founder of Yang TC) and modified by his descendents. The characteristics of Yang TC are: extended and natural postures, slow and even motions, light and steady movements, and curved, flowing lines of performance [1]. Classical Yang TC includes 108 posture, each training session consists of 20 min of warm up (low back and hamstrings stretching, gentle calisthenics and balance training), 24 min of TC practice, and 10 min of cool down.

The exercise intensity of TC appears very low owning to the slow speed and gentle movements during exercise. The slow exercise speed associated with TC actually increases the load on the lower limbs in crouching posture, since the poses are held for a comparatively long time. TC participants with different ages thus can adjust the postural height and duration to achieve similar relative exercise intensity. If the exercise intensity of TC is similar in different ages and gender, it means that TC suited not only for the elderly but also for the young. This chapter reviews the exercise intensity of TC based on existing literature, and introduces HR responses during Yang TC practice in different age and gender groups.

HR Responses in Different TC

Previous studies indicated that the exercise intensity of TC varies among different styles [13–16]. Zhou and associates [16] reported a heart rate of 134 bpm in 11 young men while practicing classical Yang TC. As for the older subjects, we have previously reported that the mean HR of subjects aged 50 to 65 years was about 130 bpm during TC practice, and 120 bpm for subjects aged

65 to 80 years [15]. During the practice of simplified TC, Gong et al. [14] reported that the HR in subjects aged 48 to 80 was only 104 bpm. The data indicates that the exercise intensity of simplified TC is lower than that of classical TC. This is likely owing to that the simplified form comprises fewer postures and excludes strenuous movements. Brown and colleagues [13] have reported that the mean HR of six young men was only 117 bpm while performing Yang TC. However, they only collected variables at 7, 14, and 21 minutes during TC practice, and the HR might drop while measuring the data. We believe that continuous monitoring of HR and $\dot{V}O_2$ is more appropriate to determine the exercise intensity of TC.

HR responses and $\dot{V}O_2$ during Yang TC Practice

In a previous study [17], we monitored the HR responses and $\dot{V}O_2$ during TC practice in 15 male TC practitioners by using the K4 telemetry equipment. The K4 system contains an O_2 and CO_2 electrode and weighs only 850 g, so it will not hinder movement of TC. To determine the blood lactate level, venous blood samples were taken before TC practice, at 1, 3, and 5 min after exercise, thus avoiding any interference with the TC practice.

Additionally, a maximal bicycle exercise testing with sequential blood lactate analysis was conducted for all subjects. At the peak exercise, the mean peak HR of subjects was 186 ± 8 bpm, and the $\dot{V}O_{2peak}$ was 39.1 ± 7.7 ml · kg^{-1} · min^{-1}. At the ventilatory threshold (VeT), subjects' HR was 135 ± 9 bpm, and the $\dot{V}O_2$ was 22.5 ± 3.3 ml · kg^{-1} · min^{-1}. During the TC practice, the mean HR was 140 ± 10 bpm and the $\dot{V}O_2$ was 21.4 ± 1.5 ml · kg^{-1} · min^{-1}. Compared with the data obtained during the exercise testing, the HR while performing TC was 58% of subjects' heart rate reserve, and the $\dot{V}O_2$ while performing TC was 55% of subjects' $\dot{V}O_{2peak}$, and this intensity was close to the ventilatory threshold. The blood lactate concentration was 3.8 mM on termination of TC, and it approximated the onset of lactate accumulation (OBLA). Because the VeT and OBLA implies the maximum exercise intensity a person can sustain over a prolonged period, the exercise intensity during TC practice appears appropriate to enhance cardiorespiratory fitness.

Figure 1 illustrates the heart rate responses during the TC practice. During the performance of TC, subjects' HR increased rapidly during the first 12 min, and then increased slowly towards the end of exercise. Figure 2 illustrates the evolution of $\dot{V}O_2$ during the TC practice. Subjects' $\dot{V}O_2$ demonstrated a sharp increase in the first three minutes, and then it achieved a steady-state towards the end of exercise.

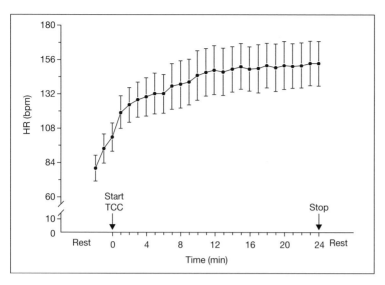

Fig. 1. The heart rate responses during TC practice (values are mean ± SD). Subjects' HR increased steadily during the first 12 min, and then it achieved a near steady-state toward the end of exercise. (Am J Chin Med 2001;29:403–410, with permission.)

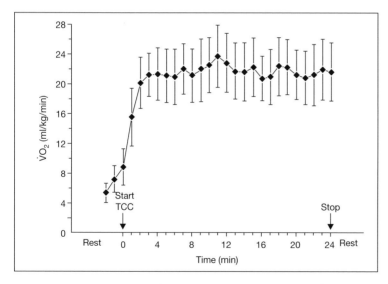

Fig. 2. The evolution of $\dot{V}O_2$ during TC practice. Subjects' $\dot{V}O_2$ showed a fast increase in the first three minutes, and then it remained at a steady-state toward the end of exercise. (Am J Chin Med 2001;29:403–410, with permission.)

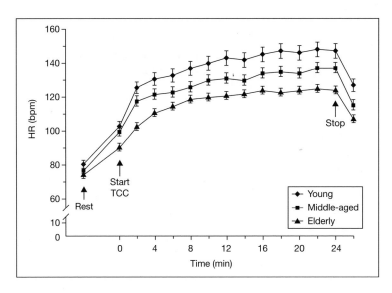

Fig. 3. Heart rate responses of men during TC practice in different age groups (◆ young group, ■ middle-aged group, ▲ elderly group, values are mean ± SE). (Am J Chin Med 2004;32:151–160, with permission.)

TC in Different Age and Gender

In a recent study [18], we measured the HR response during TC practice in 100 subjects (54 men and 46 women). They were divided into three age groups: young (25–44 y/o), middle-aged (45–64 y/o) and elderly (65–80 y/o). HR responses were continuously monitored during TC practice. In addition, each subject underwent an exercise test to determine their maximal cardiorespiratory fitness. The exercise intensity of TC was determined by comparing HR measurements obtained during the TC practice and exercise testing. Since heart rate response to the same workload varies individually, the exercise intensity is best expressed as an percentage of individual HRR.

While performing TC, subjects' HR responses were shown in figure 3 and 4. During the nearly steady state of TC practice, the mean HR of the young group was 141 ± 12 bpm in men and 136 ± 10 bpm in women, and that of the middle-aged group was 132 ± 9 bpm in men and 126 ± 11 bpm in women. In the elderly group, the mean HR was 120 ± 10 bpm in men and 115 ± 12 bpm in women. Compared with the data obtained during the exercise testing, the mean HR of men during TC practice was 57.8 ± 3.7, 56.6 ± 3.4

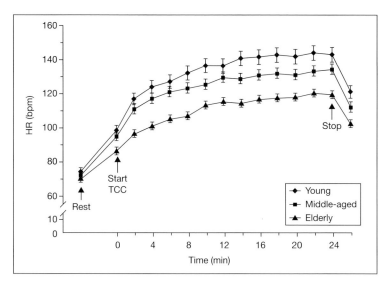

Fig. 4. Heart rate responses of women during TC practice in different age groups (◆ young group, ■ middle-aged group, ▲ elderly group, values are mean ± SE). (Am J Chin Med 2004;32:151–160, with permission.)

and 55.1 ± 3.1% of HRR in the young, middle-aged, and elderly groups, respectively. In women, the mean HR during TC was 52.7 ± 2.8, 51.5 ± 2.6, and 50.3 ± 2.9% of HRR in the three corresponding groups. The results showed the relative exercise intensity of TC was similar across different ages in each gender.

Exercise intensity and duration determine the total caloric expenditure during a training session, and thus determine the training effect. Further, load and speed of exercise determine the exercise intensity. Notably, high-intensity exercises are generally performed at a high speed. However, the training principle of traditional Chinese exercises departs from the above assumption of an association between speed and exercise intensity. TC is performed in a semi-squat posture, thus placing significant load on the lower extremities. Therefore, high-squat posture and short training duration are suited for older or unfit participants; low-squat posture and long duration are suited for younger participants. TC participants with different ages thus can adjust the exercise posture and duration to achieve a suitable level of intensity during training.

TCC has several unique characteristics. First, the slower the motion, the greater the load placed on the lower extremities. Second, the lower the posture, the greater the strength demanded. Third, most TCC motions are performed in close-chain kinematics, and thus prevent excessive stress on the joints of the lower extremities. Therefore, TCC can be safely practiced even in patients with knee arthritis [19]. The exercise mode, intensity, duration and frequency of TCC fulfill the recommendations of the American College of Sports Medicine [20] for exercise to develop and maintain cardiorespiratory fitness.

In conclusion, TC is an exercise with moderate intensity, and is aerobic in nature. The exercise intensity of TC is suitable for participants of different ages and gender to improve their functional capacity.

References

1   China Sports. Simplified 'Taijiquan', ed 2. Beijing: China Publications Center, 1983, pp 1–5.
2   Chen KM, Snyder M, Krichbaum K: Clinical use of tai chi in elderly populations. Geriatr Nurs 2001;22:198–200.
3   Lan C, Lai JS, Chen SY, Wong MK: 12-month Tai Chi training in the elderly: its effect on health fitness. Med Sci Sports Exerc 1998;30:345–351.
4   Lan C, Lai JS, Chen SY: Tai Chi Chuan: an ancient wisdom on exercise and health promotion. Sports Med 2002;32:217–224.
5   Jacobson BH, Chen HC, Cashel C, Guerrero L: The effect of T'ai Chi Chuan training on balance, kinesthetic sense, and strength. Percept Mot Skills 1997;84:27–33.
6   Wang JS, Lan C, Wong MK: Tai Chi Chuan training to enhance microcirculatory function in healthy elderly men. Arch Phys Med Rehabil 2001;82:1176–1180.
7   Wang JS, Lan C, Chen SY, Wong MK: Tai Chi Chuan training is associated with enhanced endothelium-dependent dilation in skin vasculature of healthy older men. J Am Geriatr Soc 2002; 50:1024–1030.
8   Thornton EW, Sykes KS, Tang WK: Health benefits of Tai Chi exercise: improved balance and blood pressure in middle-aged women. Health Promot Int 2004;19:33–38.
9   Kutner NG, Barnhart H, Wolf SL, McNeely E, Xu T: Self-report benefits of Tai Chi practice by older adults. J Gerontol B Psychol Sci Soc Sci 1997;52:242–246.
10 Jin P: Efficacy of Tai Chi, brisk walking, meditation, and reading in reducing mental and emotional stress. J Psychosom Res 1992;36:361–370.
11 Wolf SL, Barnhart HX, Kutner NG, et al: Reducing frailty and falls in older persons: an investigation of Tai Chi and computerized balance training. Atlanta FICSIT Group. Frailty and Injuries: Cooperative Studies of Intervention Techniques. J Am Geriatr Soc 1996;44:489–497.
12 Young DR, Appel LJ, Jee S, Miller ER: The effects of aerobic exercise and T'ai Chi on blood pressure in older people: results of a randomized trial. J Am Geriatr Soc 1999;47:277–284.
13 Brown DD, Mucci WG, Hetzler RK, Knowlton RG: Cardiovascular and ventilatory responses during formalized T'ai Chi Chuan exercise. Res Q Exerc Sport 1989;60:246–250.
14 Gong LS, Qian JA, Zhang JS, et al: Changes in heart rate and electrocardiogram during taijiquan exercise: analysis by telemetry in 100 subjects. Chin Med J 1981;94:589–592.
15 Lan C, Lai JS, Wong MK, Yu ML: Cardiorespiratory function, flexibility, and body composition among geriatric Tai Chi Chuan practitioners. Arch Phys Med Rehabil 1996;77:612–616.
16 Zhuo D, Shephard RJ, Plyley MJ, Davis GM: Cardiorespiratory and metabolic responses during Tai Chi Chuan exercise. Can J Appl Sport Sci 1984;9:7–10.
17 Lan C, Chen SY, Lai JS, Wong MK: Heart rate responses and oxygen consumption during Tai Chi Chuan practice. Am J Chin Med 2001;29:403–410.
18 Lan C, Chen SY, Lai JS: Relative exercise intensity of Tai Chi Chuan is similar in different ages and gender. Am J Chin Med 2004;32:151–160.

19 Hartman CA, Manos TM, Winter C, et al: Effects of T'ai Chi training on function and quality of life indicators in older adults with osteoarthritis. J Am Geriatr Soc 2000;48:1553–1559.
20 American College of Sports Medicine Position Stand. The recommended quantity and quality of exercise for developing and maintaining cardiorespiratory and muscular fitness, and flexibility in healthy adults. Med Sci Sports Exerc 1998;30:975–991.

Ching Lan, MD
Department of Physical Medicine and Rehabilitation, National Taiwan University Hospital
7, Chung-Shan South Road
Taipei 10016 (Taiwan)
Tel. +886 2 312 3456, Ext. 6760, Fax +886 2 2383 2834, E-Mail clan@ntu.edu.tw

Hong Y (ed): Tai Chi Chuan. State of the Art in International Research.
Med Sport Sci. Basel, Karger, 2008, vol 52, pp 20–29

··························

Tai Chi Exercise and Muscle Strength and Endurance in Older People

Dong Qing Xu[a,b], *Youlian Hong*[a], *Jing Xian Li*[a,c]

[a]Department of Sports Science and Physical Education, The Chinese University of Hong Kong, Hong Kong, [b]Department of Health and Exercise Science, Tianjin University of Sports, Tianjin, China; [c]School of Human Kinetics, University of Ottawa, Ottawa, Canada

---

Abstract

The purpose of the study was to investigate the influence of regular Tai Chi (TC) practice on muscle strength and endurance of the lower extremities in older people. Twenty-one long-term older TC practitioners were compared with 18 regular older joggers and 22 sedentary counterparts. Maximum concentric strength of knee flexors and extensors was tested at angular velocities of 30° and 120°/s. Ankle dorsiflexors and plantar flexors were tested at 30°/s. Moreover the dynamic endurance of the knee flexors and extensors was assessed at the speed of 180°/s. The strength of knee extensors and flexors in the sedentary group was significantly lower than that in the jogging group and marginally lower than that in the TC group at the higher velocity. For ankle joint, the subjects in both the TC group and the jogging group generated more torque in their ankle dorsiflexors. In addition, the muscle endurance of knee extensors was more pronounced in TC practitioners than the controls. Regular older TC practitioners and joggers showed better scores than the sedentary controls on most of the muscle strength and endurance measures. However, the magnitude of the exercise effects on muscles might depend on the characteristics of different types of exercise.

Copyright © 2008 S. Karger AG, Basel

Tai Chi (TC) is an ancient Chinese conditioning exercise. Its non-vigorous and gentle movements are suitable for older people. Regular TC practicing can produce beneficial effects on health, particularly on the maintenance of postural control in the old people [1, 2]. TC is thought to be beneficial for fall prevention in the elderly because its movements incorporate the elements of postural muscle strengthening, balance, postural alignment and concentration [3]. TC is performed in a semi-squat posture that can place a large load on the muscles of the lower extremities. The movements demand guided motions of the hip, knee and ankle joints in various directions, requiring concentric and eccentric contractions of the hip, knee and ankle muscles. These movements are similar to resistance exercises such as lunges, knee bends and squats, in terms of the degrees of hip and knee flexion and extension that are required [4]. Indeed, several studies have reported the benefits of TC exercise on muscle strength. Jacobson et al. [4] found significant improvements in the isometric strength of knee extensors after a 12-week TC intervention. Lan et al. [5] reported that a 12-month TC program was effective in enhancing the strength of the knee joints, with a 20.3% improvement for extensors and a 15.9% improvement for flexors. Recently, Wu et al. [6] reported that people who practice TC had greater isokinetic strength of the quadriceps and a lower displacement of the foot centre of pressure. Moreover, the authors showed that there was a good correlation between the eccentric strength of the knee extensors and the centre of pressure displacement. They pointed out that the maintenance of the eccentric strength of the postural muscles through the long-term practice of TC is beneficial for maintaining good postural control.

Even though TC practice is effective in the improvement of muscle strength in the old people, the related information is not complete. Firstly, declines in muscular strength, particularly ankle strength, have been associated with falls amongst the elderly [7, 8]. To date, assessments of TC exercise on muscle strength have only focused on knee extensors or flexors. Little has been mentioned about the effects on the muscles of the ankle joint. Secondly, there is a lack of comparison with other common physical activities. Regularly scheduled physical activity definitely promotes muscle function, but the effects of exercise on muscle strength are not identical due to the different exercise forms, intensity or duration. Hence, the study described herein measured the isokinetic strength of the knee and ankle joints, and knee muscle endurance amongst long-term TC practitioners, long-term jogging exercisers and their sedentary counterparts. Jogging is one of the most common forms of exercise in older people, and was thus selected as a contrast to TC exercise. The purpose of this study was to more comprehensively understand the effect of TC exercise on muscle function in the older people.

Methods

Subjects

Subjects were recruited by means of a questionnaire with a complementary interview about their physical and sporting activities (exercise experience, average exercise frequency, and duration of each exercise session). The universal inclusion criteria for all groups were (a) age 60 years or over; (b) predominantly healthy and with no history of significant cardiovascular, pulmonary, metabolic, musculoskeletal or neurological diseases; (c) no use of specific

Table 1. Demographics of subjects in the three groups (mean ± SD)

	TC group (n = 21)	Jogging group (n = 18)	Control group (n = 22)
Gender, M/F	13/8	11/7	12/10
Age, years	66.2 ± 5.1	65.2 ± 3.0	64.9 ± 3.2
Height, cm	163.6 ± 7.9	164.1 ± 9.0	164.1 ± 7.9
Weight, kg	64.8 ± 10.0	66.1 ± 13.4	69.5 ± 10.8

medications known to impair balance or strength; (d) independent living in the community with a normally active lifestyle. TC practitioners came from three clubs, where hundreds of people practice TC in a group everyday. The practices were instructed by qualified TC masters. Joggers were recruited from a large health center for older people where active individuals participate in regular exercise programs. The old subjects who participated in the sedentary control group were recruited from a large housing estate in the city. From the assessment of the collected information, a total of 61 old people were recruited in this study. The TC group was composed of 21 subjects with 4 or more years of TC experience. They regularly practiced Yang style TC every day for approximately 60 min, but were not involved in any other regular physical activity. The practice session consisted of a warm-up stretching exercise (about 8 min), a complete TC practice, and a cool-down exercise (about 7 min). The jogging group included 18 older people who had engaged in at least one hour of jogging exercise per day during the past 4 years or more (including approximately 15 min of warm-up and cool-down). The average distance of jogging was 7.9 km each time and the average jogging speed was 8.6 km/h. The joggers occasionally performed other physical activities (swimming and bicycling), but had no TC experience. The sedentary controls practiced no regular exercise for more than 5 years. An informed consent form was given to each subject before participation. The study was approved by the local medical ethics committee. No significant difference was noted in age, body height, body weight and ratio of gender across the three groups (table 1).

Testing Protocol

The testing was divided into two parts. The first assessed the strength and endurance of knee extensors and flexors. Then, after 20 min of relaxation, the strength of ankle dorsiflexors and plantar flexors was evaluated. All tests were performed on each subject's dominant leg.

A submaximal warm-up exercise (50–60 W) was performed on a bicycle ergometer (Monark, Varberg, Sweden) for 5 min before muscle tests. The Cybex Norm isokinetic dynamometer system (Cybex Corporation, USA) was used to measure the torque and work produced by specific muscle groups.

Knee Joint

The subjects sat on the examination chair with a hip angle of 90°, stabilized with the straps around the thigh being tested, as well as around the abdomen and thorax. The axis of the tested knee was aligned with the rotation axis of the dynamometer, and the lower leg was attached to the lever arm of the dynamometer. Isokinetic strength was measured using preset angular velocities of 30° and 120°/s of concentric actions for knee flexors and extensors at full available range of motion. Three maximal contractions were measured and the highest peak torque (PT) was reported. A 1.5-min rest period was allowed between the two sets of data collection at the different velocities. All torque data were normalized per kilogram of body weight for analyses (PT%).

After 3 min of relaxation on the bicycle ergometer, the dynamic endurance of the knee extensors and flexors was assessed from a recording of 40 repeated maximum isokinetic contractions with an angular velocity of 180°/s. Subjects were instructed to push and pull 'as hard and as fast as possible' in every single movement. The work expended by a knee angular motion of 10–80° was recorded. The endurance index (EI) was defined as the ratio of the work during the last five contractions over the first five contractions.

Ankle Joint

In performing isokinetic ankle dorsiflexion and plantarflexion, the subjects were positioned lying supine, with the foot attached to a footplate and fixed with two belts. The ankle joint was aligned with the axis of the dynamometer. The isokinetic contractions were performed at an angular velocity of 30°/s. Before testing, each person performed a warm-up exercise of three submaximal repetitions to familiarize themselves with the equipment. For the isokinetic test, the subjects were instructed to push the foot away from them and pull it towards them at maximum velocity through the full available range of motion for each repetition. PT was determined as the highest torque generated from the three trials, and the PT% data were analyzed.

Data Analysis

All variables were presented as means and standard deviations. One-way analysis of variance was used to determine significant differences amongst the groups. Post-hoc Tukey tests were performed when necessary to isolate the differences and p ≤ 0.05 was considered to be statistically significant.

Results

Knee Joint

The mean concentric PT% of knee flexors and extensors at the velocity of 30°/s in TC and jogging subjects showed a clear trend for being greater than those in the control group, although the differences did not reach significant levels (p = 0.058 for knee flexors, p = 0.165 for knee extensors). The differences in muscle strength amongst the three groups were significant at the velocity of 120°/s (p = 0.001 for knee flexors, p = 0.003 for knee extensors). Post-hoc comparisons indicated that the concentric strengths of knee extensors and flexors in the control group were significantly lower than those in the jogging group (p = 0.001 for flexors, p = 0.003 for extensors) and marginally

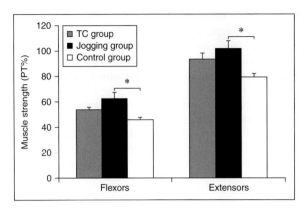

Fig. 1. Knee joint muscle strength at an angular velocity of 120°/s. Error bars indicate SEM. *p < 0.05.

lower than those in the TC group (p = 0.09 for flexors, p = 0.06 for extensors; fig. 1). No significant differences in knee muscle strength were found between the TC and jogging groups.

Ankle Joint

The PT% of dorsiflexors significantly differed amongst the three groups (p = 0.012), whereas that of plantarflexors did not (p = 0.077). Further comparisons showed that the subjects in both the TC group (p = 0.029) and the jogging group (p = 0.027) generated more torque in their ankle dorsiflexors. No significant differences in the PT% of ankle dorsiflexors and plantar flexors were observed between the TC and jogging groups (fig. 2).

Muscle Endurance

All of the subjects were able to perform the 40 maneuvers at the velocity of 180°/s. As the EI is the ratio of the work during the last 5 contractions over the first 5 contractions, a larger index reflects a greater resistance to fatigue. For knee extensors, the TC subjects demonstrated a significantly greater EI than did the sedentary controls (p = 0.027), thus indicating a better ability to maintain a higher torque level throughout the 40 contractions. The mean value of EI in the jogging group was greater than that in the control group, and slightly lower than that in the TC group, but the differences were not significant. Similar data were

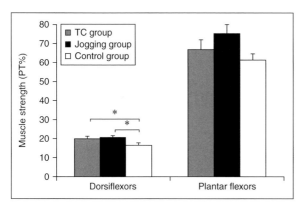

Fig. 2. Ankle muscle strength at an angular velocity of 30°/s. Error bars indicate SEM. *p < 0.05.

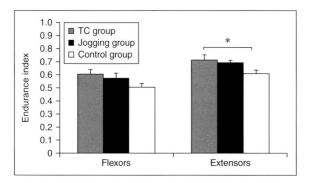

Fig. 3. EI of knee flexors and extensors at an angular velocity of 180°/s. Error bars indicate SEM. *p < 0.05.

noted for the knee flexors: the TC group displayed the best EI, the jogging group displaced the second best and the control group showed the worst EI, although the differences between the groups were not significant (fig. 3).

Discussion

As predicted, long-term regular exercisers scored or tended to score better than the sedentary controls on most of the muscle strength and endurance measures. However, the magnitude of the exercise effects on each muscle was not identical in different types of exercise. The regular joggers were much stronger than the controls in the ankle dorsiflexors, and knee flexors and extensors at high contractile speed, whereas significant effects of TC exercise were only seen in the ankle dorsiflexors. However, the muscle endurance of knee extensors was more pronounced in the TC practitioners than in the controls.

There is little doubt that muscles weaken as an individual grows old, with dynamic strength being compromised to a greater extent than isometric strength [9, 10]. Fortunately, many studies have indicated that older people adapt to resistive and endurance exercise training in a similar fashion to young people, and the decline in the metabolic and force-producing capacity of muscles can no longer be considered as an inevitable consequence of the ageing process [11]. Old people who have maintained a physically active lifestyle have demonstrated better muscle strength and endurance than their age-matched less active peers. Laforest et al. [12] reported that elderly regular tennis players had greater knee muscle strength at both low and high contractile speeds than their sedentary peers, so also was the endurance of knee extensors. It seems that our data are not very consistent with these findings. However, it should be noted that almost all of these cross-sectional studies carried out comparisons between active and inactive people. Few studies have considered the possible effects of different forms of exercise. When we individually compared the differences in muscle strength and endurance between the TC practitioners and the controls, and between the joggers and the controls, using an independent t test, the results were similar to those of most related studies. Almost all muscle strength parameters in the exercisers were significantly better than those in their sedentary counterparts, except for plantarflexor strength in the TC group and the endurance of knee flexors in the jogging group. Hence, we believe that our results might be a function of the characteristics of the specific forms of exercise. TC combines deep diaphragmatic breathing and relation with slow, gentle movements, both isometric and isotonic. Participants step with full weight on both lower extremities in a semi-squatting posture, but the heel strike is gentler than in walking because of slow and deliberate foot placement [13]. Thus, TC is regarded as low-impact and low-velocity exercise [14]. Comparatively, both TC and jogging use body weight as resistance, but jogging should produce more vigorous impact on the lower extremities than TC from their respective characteristics of exercise. Our results are similar to those of Gauchard et al. [15]. The authors compared the muscular strength of old subjects who regularly practiced proprioceptive (yoga and soft gymnastics) or bioenergetic (jogging, swimming and cycling) physical activities, and controls. The bioenergetic group showed the best muscular strength and power in the ankle and knee joints, and the proprioceptive group had average values. The authors specially mentioned that the ritual motions of Tai Chi also constituted proprioceptive exercise.

Amongst the four muscle groups of the lower extremities, TC practice stimulated significantly greater gains than in the controls in only the ankle dorsiflexors. This might be because the movements of ankle dorsiflexion are particularly emphasized in almost all forms of TC, such as slowly raising and lowering the toes under tension, dorsiflexed foot turn left or right, and so on. Exercises always give priority to improving the function of the specific muscle groups used in the exercise. Balance is influenced by strength in the muscles that control the ankle, knee and hip, which are used in the production of postural movements and gait [16]. Of particular importance is that the loss of strength in the dorsiflexor muscles is associated with falls and with difficulty in performing certain activities of daily living [7, 17]. Whipple et al. [8] reported that at the higher, more functional limb velocities, ankle weakness, particularly that which involves the dorsiflexors, appears to be an important factor underlying poor balance. Obviously, the maintenance of dorsiflexor strength in the long-term TC practitioners and joggers is likely to be beneficial for proper postural control.

Another interesting finding is that significant effects of jogging exercise on knee muscle strength were only visible at higher velocity. Rogers and Evans [11] suggested that the preferential loss and/or atrophy of fast-twitch fibers (type II) is associated with ageing. The older have fewer, but on average larger and slower, motor units [18]. A relatively greater decrease in torque with increasing speeds was thus characteristic of knee extensors in older subjects [12, 19]. As demonstrated in the present study, jogging seems to counteract this impairment. This might be very important for the older because high-speed muscle contraction is necessary for them to maintain function in daily activities, such as normal walking speed and timely response to perturbation.

Increased muscle endurance might be of great practical importance to the older as a means of reducing the increased risk of accidents and falling. Muscle endurance depends on the ability to transport oxygen to active muscles (cardiovascular factors) and the ability of muscles to use the oxygen supplied (intrinsic muscular biochemical factors) [11, 20]. In our study, TC practitioners achieved the best scores on muscle endurance. TC movements are slow, continuous, smooth and well controlled and have been regarded as a low-intensity aerobic activity by some researchers [21]. From the characteristics of TC movement, TC exercise involves the use of slow-twitch muscle fibers which, when trained, have a higher concentration of myoglobin, a larger number of capillaries and a higher content of mitochondria and thus mitochondrial enzymes, than fast-twitch fibers. These factors enable the slow-twitch fibers to have a high resistance to fatigue due to their high capacity for aerobic metabolism. It is through this training response that regular TC exercise could improve muscle endurance.

Conclusion

Our study confirmed that regular physical activity could produce positive effects on muscle function. Although the benefits of the long-term TC practice on muscle strength in the lower extremity did not seem superior to those of long-term jogging, the maintenance of dorsiflexion strength and knee extension endurance in TC practitioners might be of practical importance for older people in everyday life.

Acknowledgements

The work described in this paper was fully supported by a grant from the Research Grants Council of the Hong Kong Special Administrative Region (project CUHK4360/00H).

References

1   Hong Y, Li JX, Robinson PD: Balance control, flexibility, and cardiorespiratory fitness among older Tai Chi practitioners. Br J Sports Med 2000;34:29–34.
2   Tse SK, Bailey DM: T'ai chi and postural control in the well elderly. Am J Occup Thera 1992;46:295–300.
3   Wolf SL, Barnhart HX, Kutner NG, McNeely E, Coogler C, Xu T: Reducing frailty and falls in older persons: an investigation of Tai Chi and computerized balance training. J Am Geriatr Soc 1996;44:489–497.
4   Jacobson BH, Chen HC, Cashel C, Guerrero L: The effect of Tai Chi Chuan training on balance, kinesthetic sense, and strength. Percept Mot Skills 1997;84:27–33.
5   Lan C, Lai JS, Chen SY, Wong MK: 12-month Tai Chi training in the elderly: its effect on health fitness. Med Sci Sports Exerc 1998;30:345–351.
6   Wu G, Zhao F, Zhou X, Wei L: Improvement of isokinetic knee extensor strength and reduction of postural sway in the elderly from long-term Tai Chi. Arch Phys Med Rehabil 2002;83:1364–1369.
7   Fiatarone M, Evans W: The etiology and reversibility of muscle dysfunction in the aged. J Gerontol 1993;48:77–83.
8   Whipple RH, Wolfson LI, Amerman PM: The relationship of knee and ankle weakness to falls in nursing home residents: An isokinetic study. J Am Geriatr Soc 1987;35:13–20.
9   Davies CT, Thomas DO, White MJ: Mechanical properties of young and elderly human muscle. Acta Med Scand Suppl 1986;711:219–226.
10 Pearson MB, Bassey EJ, Bendall MJ: The effects of age on muscle strength and anthropometric indices within a group of elderly men and women. Age Ageing 1985;14:230–234.
11 Rogers MA, Evans WJ: Changes in skeletal muscle with aging: effects of exercise training. Exerc Sport Sci Rev 1993;21:65–102.
12 Laforest S, St-Pierre DMM, Cyr J, Gayton D: Effects of age and regular exercise on muscle strength and endurance. Eur J Appl Physiol 1990;60:104–111.
13 Kirsteins AE, Dietz F, Hwang SM: Evaluating the safety and potential use of a weight-bearing exercise, Tai-Chi Chuan, for reheumatoid arthritis patients. Am J Phys Med Rehabil 1991;70:136–141.
14 Lan C, Lai JS, Chen SY: Tai Chi Chuan to improve muscular strength and endurance in elderly individuals: a pilot study. Arch Phys Med Rehabil 2000;81:604–607.

15 Gauchard G, Jeandel C, Tessier A, Perrin PP: Beneficial effect of proprioceptive physical activities on balance control in elderly human subjects. Neurosci Lett 1999;273:81–84.
16 Dayhoff NE, Suhrheinrich J, Wigglesworth J, Topp R, Moore S: Balance and muscle strength as predictors of frailty among older adults. J Gerontol Nurs 1998;24:18–27; quiz 54–55.
17 Tinetti ME, Speechley M, Ginter SF: Risk factors for falls among elderly persons living in the community. New Engl J Med 1988;319:1190–1193.
18 Rice CL, Cunningham DA, Paterson DH, Dickinson JR: Strength training alters contractile properties of the triceps brachii in men aged 65–78 years. Eur J Appl Physiol 1993;66:275–280.
19 Larsson L, Grimby G, Karlsson J: Muscle strength and speed of movement in relation to age and muscle morphology. J Appl Physiol 1979;46:451–456.
20 Gersten JW: Effect of exercise on muscle function decline with aging. West J Med 1991;154: 579–582.
21 Brown DD, Mucci WG, Hetzler RK, Knowlton RG: Cardiovascular and ventilatory responses during formalized T'ai Chi Chuan exercise. Res Q Exerc Sport 1989;60:246–250.

Dong Qing Xu, PhD
Department of Health and Exercise Science
Tianjin University of Sports
Tianjin (China)
Tel. +86 22 23012459, E-Mail xudongqing54@yahoo.com.cn

Hong Y (ed): Tai Chi Chuan. State of the Art in International Research.
Med Sport Sci. Basel, Karger, 2008, vol 52, pp 30–39

....

Muscle Action Pattern and Knee Extensor Strength of Older Tai Chi Exercisers

Ge Wu

Department of Rehabilitation and Movement Science,
The University of Vermont, Burlington, VT., USA

Abstract

Background/Aims: Tai Chi (TC) practice has been shown to improve leg muscle strength among elders. This study examined the leg muscle action patterns during a typical TC movement, and their relationship with knee extensor strength and knee flexion angle in single leg stance. **Methods:** Surface electromyography of four leg muscles and knee movement were recorded from 5 female elderly TC practitioners while performing a TC movement and normal walking, respectively. The Maximum knee extensor strength was also measured. The duration and magnitude of electromyography were compared between the TC movement and walking, and were correlated with the knee extensor strength and knee flexion angle. **Results:** Ankle dorsiflexors and knee extensors were activated significantly longer and higher during the TC movement than during walking. The duration and magnitude of all four leg muscles during the TC movement were positively correlated with the knee extensor strength and knee flexion angle, and these correlations were stronger than during walking. **Conclusion:** The TC movement puts more demand on ankle dorsiflexors and knee extensors that are not otherwise heavily recruited during walking. The degree of knee flexion during single leg stance of the TC movement may be a key element for improving leg muscle strength.

It has been well demonstrated that long-term Tai Chi (TC) exercises improve leg muscle strength, especially knee extensors among elders [1–4]. Cross-sectional studies have shown that long-term elderly TC practitioners have significantly stronger knee extensors than non-TC practitioners [4]. Even after a few months of regular practice of TC, elders are shown to increase their knee extensor strength and endurance significantly more than those who do not practice TC [1–3].

The positive effect of TC exercise on leg muscle strength may be related to the unique kinematic and kinetic features of TC movements. In principle, TC movements are performed with a crouched leg posture throughout, including both double and single leg stances. The crouched leg posture and wide base of support place a high demand on ankle dorsiflexors and knee extensors [5]. Thus, a long-term practice of these TC movements would evidently lead to the strengthening of these muscles.

However, maintaining a couched leg posture, especially during single leg stance, is not an easy task. For elders, this posture is even more challenging because of their decreased muscle strength, a normal consequence of aging [6]. Do elders practice TC with the crouched leg posture? Is the rigor of the crouched leg posture related to the leg muscle strength? What are the muscle action patterns during TC movements? Are they also related to leg muscle strength?

The goal of this study was to examine muscle action patterns of elderly TC practitioners during TC movement, and their relationship with leg posture and knee extensor strength. It was hypothesized that (1) elderly TC practitioners would have longer duration and higher level ankle dorsiflexor and knee extensor activations during TC movement than during normal walking, and (2) the duration and magnitude of these muscle actions are correlated with the knee extensor strength and knee flexion angle during TC movement.

To test these hypotheses, surface electromyography (EMG) of four leg muscles and joint movement of ankle and knee were recorded from a group of elderly TC practitioners while performing a TC movement, Parting the Wild Horse Mane, and normal walking. The leg movement of the Parting the Wild Horse Mane is a typical leg posture used in more than 64% of the movements in a simplified TC form, and more than 55% in a complete Yang style TC form [7]. It is a cyclic motion of the lower extremities, with a well-defined sequence and timing that are similar to that of normal walking. These similarities make it possible to carry out a comparison between this TC movement and normal walking, a popular exercise among elders. Maximum knee extensor strength was also measured and was correlated with muscle action patterns and knee joint angle.

Methods

Subjects

Five female volunteers aged 61–84 (mean age 72.6 ± 8.7) years participated in the study. Their average height and weight were 156 ± 10 cm and 66 ± 12 kg, respectively. They were recruited on a voluntary basis from TC exercise programs in the local area, and had been practicing Yang style TC regularly for the past 15 weeks. They had no presence of any of the following: vestibular dysfunction, cardiovascular disease, musculoskeletal disorders, recent lower extremity fracture or sprain in the past 6 months, or current joint pain that prevented normal functioning in the ankle, knee and hip joints. All subjects signed an approved informed consent form prior to testing.

Equipment

Silver/silver chloride bipolar surface EMG electrodes (Myotronics-Noromed, Inc., Tukwila, Wash., USA) were used to record EMG activities of leg muscles. The surface of each electrode (0.8 mm in diameter) contained a gel-like substance to ensure conduction quality of the EMG signal. The EMG signal from each electrode was band-pass filtered by a two-stage amplifier (Elite, Bioengineering Technology and Systems, Milan, Italy) with a frequency range of 10–200 Hz and was integrated with a time constant of 5 s. The amplifier gain was adjusted such that the EMG signal from the maximum voluntary contraction of each muscle was not saturated.

A set of three 50 Hz infra-red sensitive cameras (Elite, Bioengineering Technology and Systems) was used to record the spatial movement of reflective markers attached to various body landmarks. The cameras were set up along the left side of an 8-meter walkway, and were calibrated prior to testing for a 2 m (height) × 2 m (length) × 1 m (depth) viewing volume according to the manufacturer's instructions.

A biomechanical force plate (Advanced Mechanical Technology Inc., Watertown, Mass., USA) was used to record the foot-floor contact force. It was embedded in the middle of the walkway. The outputs from the force plate were low pass filtered at 10.5 Hz and amplified with a gain of 2,000 by a set of amplifiers provided by the manufacturer. The amplifiers were adjusted to offset the DC shift prior to testing.

A hydraulic handheld dynamometer (Fabrication Enterprises, Inc., Irvington, N.Y., USA) was used to measure isometric knee extensor strength. The dynamometer was zeroed before testing.

The recordings of the integrated EMG, reflective marker movement, and foot-floor contact force were synchronized and collected at 50 Hz by a 64-channel, 12-bit data acquisition system (Elite, Bioengineering Technology and Systems).

Procedures

Each subject wore black spandex shorts and was seated on a plinth with the left leg flexed to 90° down the side of the plinth. The dynamometer was positioned at the anterior aspect of the lower leg above the malleoli. The subject was asked to push into the dynamometer as hard as possible for at least 5 s. Three trials were repeated. The reading from the dynamometer was recorded, along with the distance from the dynamometer to lateral femoral epicondyle.

EMG electrodes were placed on tibialis anterior (TA), soleus (SOL), rectus femoris (RF), and semitendinosus (ST) of the left leg. The location of each muscle belly was found using palpation and muscle resistance tests. The contact area was shaved, scrubbed and cleaned by alcohol wipes. A bipoloar electrode was placed parallel to the muscle fiber direction. A ground electrode was also placed on the medial side of the subject's left knee. All electrodes were connected to the first stage amplifier attached to the subject's waist, which was then connected to the second stage amplifier through a fiber optic cable.

Reflective markers (10 mm in diameter) were placed, using double adhesive tape, on the fifth metatarsal head, heel, lateral malleolus, lateral femoral epicondyle, the greater trochanter, and the anterior superior iliac spine, all on the left side of the body. One additional marker was placed on the top right corner of each force plate.

Prior to testing, each subject practiced the Parting the Wild Horse's Mane movement for 5 min. A starting position 1 was identified so that the subject was able to land the left foot on the force plate during the first cycle of the movement. Another starting position (2) was also identified for normal walking. Once ready, the subject stood at the starting position 1 and began the TC movement at a self-determined speed until the end of the first cycle. A minimum of six trials were repeated. After a brief rest period (2–3 min), the subject stood at the starting position 2 and began walking at a self-determined slow speed, for a minimum of six repetitions. The subject was barefooted and asked to keep her hands on the hips for both gaits. A calibration trial was recorded before, during and after the testing, respectively. During the calibration trial, each subject stood quietly assuming the anatomically neutral posture for 3 s.

Data Analysis

The stance phase of the left leg during the TC movement and normal walking was divided into three subphases: double stance phase I (DSI), single stance phase (SS), and double stance phase II (DSII). The timing for these subphases was determined based on the vertical foot-floor contact force profile [5]. The joint range of motion of the ankle (flexion/extension) and knee (flexion/extension) during each subphase was computed from the marker movement. The activation time (ON time) and magnitude (RMS, or root-mean square) of each muscle during each subphase were determined by the EMG recordings [5].

A one-tailed, paired t-test was used to compare the difference of each variable between the TC movement and normal waking. The difference was considered statistically significant when the p value for each comparison was less than 0.05. In addition, Pearson correlation coefficient (CC) was computed between knee extensor strength and muscle action patterns and joint range of motion. The correlation was considered significant with a p value less than 0.05.

Results

Muscle Action Patterns

The EMG trajectories of four leg muscles during both TC movement and walking are shown in figure 1. There were significant differences between the TC movement and walking in the TA and RF muscle ON time ($p < 0.049$) in all three sub-stance phases, and no significant differences in the SOL and ST muscles ($p > 0.088$; fig. 2). Both TA and RF muscles were activated significantly longer (from 3 to 33 times) during TC movement throughout the stance phase. Although the ST muscle was on average activated longer during TC movement, there was a large variation among the subjects.

There were significant differences between the TC movement and walking in the magnitude of TA, RF and SOL muscle actions during the SS phase only ($p < 0.05$; fig. 3). Both TA and RF muscles were activated at a higher magnitude during TC movement in all three sub-stance phases, with the SS phase being significantly higher. In contrast, the SOL muscle was activated at a lower

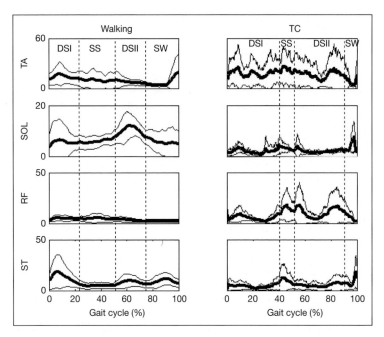

Fig. 1. Ensemble average (thick lines) and ±1 standard deviation (thin lines) of EMG signals of four leg muscles during one complete gait cycle of the TC movement and walking. The stance phases are also shown. SW = Swing.

magnitude during the TC movement throughout the three sub-stance phases, with the SS phase being significantly lower.

Correlation with Knee Extensor Strength and Knee Flexion Angle

The knee extensor strength was positively correlated with the ON time (CC = 0.71–0.97) and RMS (CC = 0.19–0.93) of all four muscles during the TC movement, with the correlation to the SOL ON time and TA and SOL RMS being statistically significant ($p < 0.05$). The correlation between knee extensor strength and muscle ON time or EMG RMS during walking was not consistent among the four muscles, with the TA and ST muscles showing positive correlations, and the SOL and RF muscles showing negative correlations, all weaker than during TC movement, and all statistically insignificant (figs 4 and 5).

There was a significant difference between the TC movement and walking in maximum knee flexion range ($p = 0.035$) during the SS phase, with the TC movement having significantly more knee flexion ($15 \pm 10°$) than walking ($8 \pm 2°$). The knee flexion angle during the SS phase was positively correlated with the ON time and RMS value of all four muscles during the TC movement

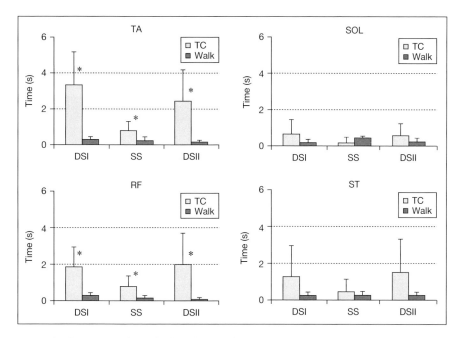

Fig. 2. Mean and standard deviation of muscle ON time during TC movement and walking in three sub-stance phases (DSI, SS and DSII). Asterisk indicates significant difference between TC movement and walking.

(table 1). It was also positively and significantly correlated with the maximum knee extensor strength during the SS phase of the TC movement (CC = 0.84), while negatively correlated during walking (CC = −0.25).

Discussion

This study aimed to examine leg muscle action patterns of elderly TC practitioners during a TC movement and their relationship with knee flexion angle and knee extensor strength. The results demonstrate that their ankle dorsiflexors and knee extensors are activated at least twice as long and as high during TC movement as during walking, and are all positively correlated with the knee flexion angle during single leg stance as well as maximum knee extensor strength.

The muscle action patterns during TC movement among the elderly TC practitioners are consistent with the literature. In an earlier study of the kinematics and EMG of leg muscles during a TC gait among healthy young adults, Wu et al. [5] have found that the TC movement involves a significantly longer

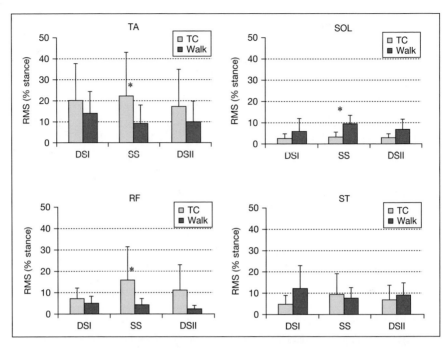

Fig. 3. Mean and standard deviation of muscle EMG magnitude (RMS) during TC movement and walking in three sub-stance phases (DSI, SS and DSII). Asterisk indicates significant difference between TC movement and walking.

Table 1. CCs of knee flexion angle during SS phase with ON time and RMS value of four leg muscles

CC	ON time		RMS	
	TC	Walk	TC	Walk
TA	0.77	0.10	0.70	0.05
SOL	0.94*	0.61	0.99*	0.73
RF	0.77	−0.03	0.19	0.31
ST	0.98*	0.71	0.76	0.60

*p < 0.05.

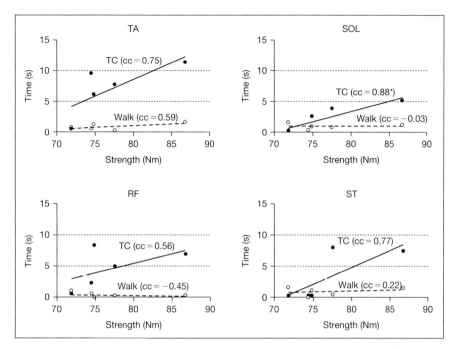

Fig. 4. Scattered and linear regression line of knee extensor strength versus muscle ON time during the entire stance phase of TC movement (filled circle and solid line) and walking (open circle and dashed line). Asterisk indicates significance of the correlation coefficient at $\alpha = 0.05$.

duration and higher magnitude of ankle dorsiflexor and knee extensor muscle actions as compared to normal gait. A kinematics and EMG analysis of the push hand movement of TCC by Chan et al. [8] have also found high levels of activation in the knee extensors.

The results from this study demonstrate that the TC movement puts more demand on the ankle dorsiflexors and knee extensors than their antagonist muscles, suggesting that the TC practice may be particularly beneficial for these muscles. Indeed, studies have shown that long-term elderly TC practitioners have significantly stronger knee extensors than nonpractitioners, but similar knee flexors [4].

Nevertheless, all muscle activities during the TC movement have demonstrated a positive correlation with the amount of knee flexion during single leg stance of the TC movement and with the knee extensor strength. Also, there is a strong and significant correlation between knee flexion and knee extensor strength. Although these correlations do not directly suggest the causal effect, the distinct contrast with the lack of correlations during walking suggests that

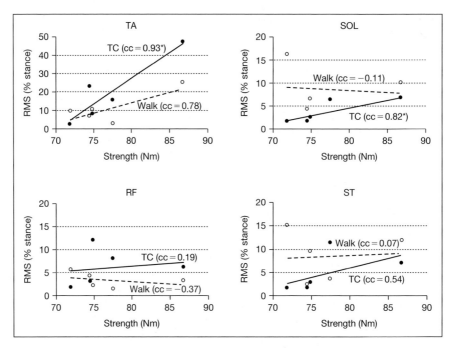

Fig. 5. Scattered and linear regression line of knee extensor strength versus muscle EMG RMS during the entire stance phase of TC movement (filled circle and solid line) and walking (open circle and dashed line). Asterisk indicates significance of the correlation coefficient at $\alpha = 0.05$.

TC practice is more demanding on leg muscles than walking. The degree of the crouched leg posture during single leg stance of a TC movement may well reflect an individual's overall muscular strength, and may be a key element for improving the strength of leg muscles.

Although the TC movement selected for testing in this study involves a basic and most popular leg posture, it, nevertheless, does not represent the entire TC movement set. Movements involving travel backward or to the side may involve different muscle action patterns. Other muscles such as abductors and trunk stabilizers may also be involved. Thus, studies that include comprehensive analysis of other muscles and other TC movements are needed in the future. Moreover, this study has compared the muscle action patterns during TC movement with those during walking. Although normal walking is a basic activity of daily living and a popular form of exercise for elders, future studies should consider comparing it with other strengthening exercises so that the effects of TC practice on muscle strength can be directly demonstrated. Finally, this study includes a relatively small sample size. The large variation in this population warrants future studies with a larger and diverse sample.

Conclusions

This study examined the muscle action patterns of elderly TC practitioners during a TC movement, Parting the Wild Horse Mane, and their relationship with leg posture and knee extensor strength. The results demonstrated significantly longer duration and higher magnitude of ankle dorsiflexor and knee extensor EMG activities during the TC movement than during walking. Also, all muscle activities during the TC movement were positively correlated with the knee flexion angle in single leg stance and maximum knee extensor strength.

Acknowledgement

This work was supported in part by the National Science Foundation, and by the University of Vermont. The author would like to thank Debra Millon for assistance in data collection and processing.

References

1   Lan C, Lai JS, Chen SY, Wong MK: Tai Chi Chuan to improve muscular strength and endurance in elderly individuals: a pilot study. Arch Phys Med Rehabil 2000;81:604–607.
2   Lan C, Lai JS, Chen SY, Wong MK: 12-month Tai Chi training in the elderly: its effect on health fitness. Med Sci Sports Exerc 1998;30:345–351.
3   Christou EA, Yang Y, Rosengren KS: Taiji training improves knee extensor strength and force control in older adults. J Gerontol A Biol Sci Med Sci 2003;58:M763–M766.
4   Wu G, Zhao F, Zhou X, Wei L: Improvement of isokinetic knee extensor strength and reduction of postural sway in the elderly from long-term Tai Chi exercise. Arch Phys Med Rehabil 2002;83: 1364–1369.
5   Wu G, Liu W, Hitt J, Millon D: Spatial, temporal and muscle action patterns of Tai Chi gait. J Electromyogr Kinesiol 2004;14:343–354.
6   Bäckman E, Johansson V, Häger B, Sjöblom P, Henriksson KG: Isometric muscle strength and muscular endurance in normal persons aged between 17 and 70 years. Scand J Rehabil Med 1995;27: 109–117.
7   Shen JZ, Gu LX: Complete Book of Tai Chi Quan (in Chinese), ed 13. China, Ren Min Ti Yu Chu Ban She, 1998.
8   Chan SP, Luk TC, Hong Y: Kinematic and electromyographic analysis of the push movement in Tai Chi. Br J Sports Med 2003;37:339–344.

Prof. Ge Wu, PhD
305 Rowell Building
Burlington, VT 05405 (USA)
Tel. +1 802 656 2556, Fax +1 802 656 6586, E-Mail ge.wu@uvm.edu

Hong Y (ed): Tai Chi Chuan. State of the Art in International Research.
Med Sport Sci. Basel, Karger, 2008, vol 52, pp 40–53

....

The Effectiveness of Tai Chi Exercise in Improving Aerobic Capacity: An Updated Meta-Analysis

Ruth E. Taylor-Piliae

College of Nursing, The University of Arizona, Tucson, Ariz., USA

Abstract

Purpose: To determine if Tai Chi exercise is effective in improving aerobic capacity. **Methods:** A computerized search of seven databases was conducted using the mesh term 'Tai Ji', published between January 1, 2000, and June 1, 2007, in order to update a previous meta-analysis examining the effect of Tai Chi on aerobic capacity. Effect sizes (ESs) and 95% confidence intervals were calculated using D-STAT software. The ES for each study was weighted by the sample size and pooled variance. The effects of Tai Chi exercise on aerobic capacity were calculated including study design, gender, age, and type of comparison group. **Results:** A total of 170 citations were obtained, with 7 new studies meeting the inclusion criteria and added to studies from the previous meta-analysis. Large significant effects of Tai Chi on aerobic capacity were found for subjects enrolled in the cross-sectional studies (ES = 1.33), in both women and men (1.09 and 0.86, respectively), among adults $\geq$55 years old (ES = 1.07), and when comparing sedentary subjects with those in Tai Chi exercise groups (ES = 0.99). Small to moderate effects, though nonsignificant, were found for subjects enrolled in the experimental studies (ES = 0.38), adults <55 years old (ES = 0.16), and when comparing subjects participating in other physical activity with those in Tai Chi exercise groups (ES = 0.45). **Conclusions:** Tai Chi exercise is effective in improving aerobic capacity when practiced long term. Middle-aged and older women and men benefit most, with greater gains seen among those initially sedentary. Tai Chi can be recommended as an alternative aerobic exercise, particularly among sedentary adults $\geq$55 years old.

In the United States, approximately 57% of adults aged 45–65 years old are not meeting the national recommendation for physical activity [1]. Regular physical activity is associated with reductions in mortality and disability from several chronic diseases, such as coronary heart disease, hypertension, diabetes, colon cancer and osteoarthritis, and improvements in physiological and psychological functioning [1, 2]. However, despite reported benefits of regular physical activity, most adults do not achieve recommended levels. The challenge and opportunity is to make physical activity more accessible to adults of all ages, interests and abilities [1, 2].

Tai Chi exercise has been practiced in China for hundreds of years, and is gaining popularity among persons in Western countries as an alternative form of exercise [3–5]. Reported benefits of Tai Chi exercise include improvements in physiological and psychological functioning such as lower blood pressure, better balance, strength and flexibility, fall prevention, improved mood and well-being, and reduced stress [6, 7]. Tai Chi is a low-impact, moderate-intensity exercise requiring approximately 4.0 metabolic equivalents to perform, which is similar in intensity to brisk walking [8].

The effectiveness of Tai Chi exercise in improving aerobic capacity is important to know, if clinicians would like to recommend Tai Chi as an alternative form of exercise. A previous meta-analysis conducted by Taylor-Piliae and Froelicher [9] was done to estimate the extent to which Tai Chi exercise affects aerobic capacity. A meta-analysis involves the integration of results from several single studies, enabling the investigator to estimate effects of treatments or interventions, and summarize the results into useful clinical information [10]. The previous meta-analysis by Taylor-Piliae and Froelicher provided preliminary evidence for aerobic benefits of Tai Chi, though it was limited by the number of studies available [9]. Since the publication of the previous meta-analysis [9], the number of research studies examining Tai Chi exercise has increased exponentially. Therefore, the purpose of this study was to update the previous meta-analysis by searching for additional recently published studies, to determine if Tai Chi exercise is effective in improving aerobic capacity.

Methods

Study Retrieval

A computerized search of seven databases (Biosis, CINAHL, Cochrane Library, Digital Dissertations, PsychINFO and PubMed) was conducted using the mesh term 'Tai Ji', to obtain studies published between January 1, 2000, through June 1, 2007. All languages were accepted. A total of 170 citations were obtained (fig. 1). Abstracts of all research studies were reviewed using a study selection form to determine if subjects were randomly assigned to a Tai Chi exercise intervention or if a Tai Chi exercise group was compared with another group; and if aerobic capacity was an outcome measure.

Following initial study review, 41 studies were examined in depth to determine if they met the inclusion criteria. A total of 7 additional studies [11–17] met the inclusion criteria and were added to the 7 studies [18–24] from the previous meta-analysis [9] for inclusion in this updated

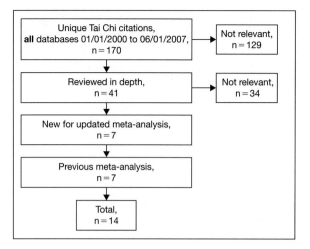

Fig. 1. Search strategy.

meta-analysis. Of the 14 studies included in this meta-analysis, there were 7 experimental studies, and 6 cross-sectional studies (tables 1 and 2, respectively). In the cross-sectional studies, 2 groups of different subjects were matched on age, gender and body composition, allowing for adequate group comparisons. Cross-sectional data from one prospective cohort study (baseline data) were also included in the analysis [14], as subjects in the study were matched at baseline on age, gender and body composition, allowing for adequate group comparisons.

Study Quality

All studies were critically appraised on a total of 16 study elements to determine a study quality score [9]. Elements reviewed included study design, sample selection, description of the independent variable (Tai Chi), description of the outcome measure (aerobic capacity), data analyses and results. Each item had a possible score of 0–2 (0 = absent, 1 = partially defined, 2 = clearly defined), with possible scores ranging from 0 to 32. The methodological quality of both experimental and cross-sectional studies could be assessed using this tool. Any study with a quality score below 67% (<21) of the total possible score [25], was set as the criteria for elimination from this analysis.

Classifying and Coding Study Characteristics

A coding form was used to abstract study data and then entered into SPSS [26] for analyses. Study characteristics abstracted included study design, intervention length and attrition for the experimental studies, years of Tai Chi for the cross-sectional studies, measurement of aerobic capacity (peak oxygen uptake), and style of Tai Chi. Type of study populations, subjects' age, gender, size of groups, and type of comparison groups (e.g. sedentary) were also abstracted.

Table 1. Experimental studies examining Tai Chi and aerobic capacity

Author/ year	Study design	Study sample/% attrition	Group	Size	Gender	Mean age in years	Tai Chi style	Length of inter- vention, weeks	Baseline mean VO$_2$ peak (ml · kg^{-1} min^{-1})	Follow-up mean VO$_2$ peak (ml · kg^{-1} min^{-1})	ES	LBCI	UBCI
Brown et al., 1995	RCT	healthy sedentary adults/25% attrition	Tai Chi	11	men	50.4 (5.7)	not specified	16	31.7 (5.1)	30.8 (4.1)	−0.36	−1.15	+0.44
			control (sedentary)	14	men	50.5 (7.4)	–		31.9 (5.4)	32.7 (5.8)			
			Tai Chi	7	women	51.5 (8.3)	not specified	16	25.0 (4.4)	23.8 (4.7)	−0.31	−1.19	+0.58
			control (sedentary)	17	women	53.6 (9.4)	–		26.7 (6.0)	25.2 (4.4)			
Lan et al., 1998	quasi- exper.	community dwelling older adults/ 13% attrition	Tai Chi	13	men	65.2 (4.2)	Yang, 108 postures	52	24.2 (5.2)	28.1 (5.4)	+0.82	−0.14	+1.78
			control (sedentary)	11	men	66.6 (3.9)	–		24.0 (4.8)	23.6 (5.0)			
			Tai Chi	15	women	64.9 (4.7)	Yang, 108 postures	52	16.0 (2.5)	19.4 (2.8)	+1.33	−0.36	+2.31
			control (sedentary)	13	women	65.4 (3.8)	–		15.8 (2.5)	15.6 (2.6)			
Lan et al., 1999	quasi- exper.	post-CABG/ 26% attrition	Tai Chi	12	men	55.7 (7.1)	Yang, 108 postures	52	26.2 (4.4)	28.9 (5.0)	+0.66	−0.25	+1.56
			control (walking program)	15	men	57.2 (7.6)	–		26.0 (3.9)	25.6 (4.6)			

Table 1. (continued)

Author/ year	Study design	Study sample/% attrition	Group	Size	Gender	Mean age in years	Tai Chi style	Length of intervention, weeks	Baseline mean VO₂ peak (ml · kg⁻¹ min⁻¹)	Follow-up mean VO₂ peak (ml · kg⁻¹ min⁻¹)	ES	LBCI	UBCI
Young et al., 1999	RCT	sedentary with HTN/ 18% attrition	Tai Chi	31	6-men 25-women	66.4 (5.1)	Yang, 13 postures	12	20.4 (3.9)	0.97 (4.1)*	−0.16	−0.71	+0.39
			control (aerobic exercise)	31	7-men 24-women	67.0 (7.9)	–		19.2 (4.5)	1.64 (4.1)*			
Song et al., 2003	RCT	Osteoarthritis/ 41% attrition	Tai Chi	38	women	64.8 (6.0)	Sun, 12 postures	12	24.1 (4.3)	1.6 (6.0)*	+0.16	−0.30	+0.63
			control (sedentary)	34	women	62.5 (5.6)	–		24.0 (4.2)	0.9 (4.2)*			
Yeh et al., 2004	RCT	chronic stable heart failure/ 0 % attrition	Tai Chi	15	10-men 5-women	66 (12)	Yang, 5 postures	12	10.5 (3.0)	11.4 (3.0)	+0.20	−0.51	+0.92
			control (usual care)	15	9-men 6-women	61 (14)	–		11.1 (6.0)	10.4 (6.0)			
Audette et al., 2006	quasi-exper.	healthy sedentary older adults/ 21% attrition	Tai Chi	11	women	71.5 (4.6)	Yang, 10 postures	12	21.6 (5.2)	4.2 (3.0)*	+1.05	+0.08	+2.02
			control (sedentary)	8	women	73.5 (5.7)	–		26.8 (8.3)	−4.4 (3.0)*			

RCT = Randomized clinical trial; quasi-exper. = quasi-experimental study; ES = effect size; LBCI = lower bound confidence interval; UBCI= upper bound confidence interval; post-CABG = post coronary artery bypass graft; HTN = hypertension; asterisk signifies mean change in aerobic capacity. Figures in parentheses indicate SD.
ES is not significant if zero is included in the confidence interval.

Table 2. Cross-sectional studies* examining Tai Chi and aerobic capacity

Author/ year	Study design	Study sample	Group	Size	Gender	Mean age years	Tai Chi style	Mean Years Tai Chi	Mean VO$_2$ peak (ml · kg^{-1} · min^{-1})	ES	LBCI	UBCI
Schneider et al., 1991	cross-sectional	martial arts practitioners	Tai Chi	10	men	35.5 (3.9)	not specified	6.8 (3.4)	44.3 (6.6)	+0.16	−0.72	+1.04
			Wing Chun	10	men	30.0 (5.0)	–		43.4 (4.0)			
Lai et al., 1993	cross-sectional	healthy adults	Tai Chi	21	men	58.7 (3.9)	Yang, 108 postures	6.3 (3.3)	33.9 (6.3)	+1.38	+0.73	+2.04
			sedentary	23	men	59.1 (4.0)	–		26.3 (4.4)			
			Tai Chi	20	women	58.3 (4.8)	Yang, 108 postures	6.3 (3.3)	21.8 (2.2)	+0.89	+0.28	+1.50
			sedentary	26	women	57.5 (4.7)	–		19.0 (3.6)			
Lai et al., 1995	prospective cohort baseline data	community dwelling older adults	Tai Chi	23	men	64.3 (7.3)	Yang, 108 postures	6.7 (3.3)	31.6 (7.6)	+1.12	+0.49	+1.76
			sedentary	21	men	63.6 (5.3)	–		24.4 (4.4)			
			Tai Chi	22	women	60.9 (4.5)	Yang, 108 postures	6.7 (3.3)	20.7 (2.3)	+1.91	+1.16	+2.67
			sedentary	18	women	62.6 (4.0)	–		16.2 (2.3)			
Lan et al., 1996	cross-sectional	community dwelling older adults	Tai Chi	22	men	70.4 (4.1)	Yang, 108 postures	11.8 (5.6)	26.9 (4.7)	+1.23	+0.55	+1.91
			sedentary	18	men	69.5 (4.2)	–		21.8 (3.1)			
			Tai Chi	19	women	66.9 (2.7)	Yang, 108 postures	11.8 (5.6)	20.1 (2.9)	+1.40	+0.67	+2.13
			sedentary	17	women	67.1 (2.8)	–		16.5 (2.0)			

Table 2. (continued)

Author/ year	Study design	Study sample	Group	Size	Gender	Mean age in year	Tai Chi style	Mean Years Tai Chi	Mean VO$_2$ peak (ml · kg^{-1} min^{-1})	ES	LBCI	UBCI
Wang et al., 2002	cross-sectional	healthy non-smokers	Tai Chi	10	women	69.9 (1.5)	Yang, 108 postures	11.2 (3.4)	23.4 (2.2)	+2.25	+1.13	+3.36
			sedentary	10	women	67.0 (1.0)	–		17.4 (2.8)			
Liu et al., 2003	cross-sectional	healthy active adults	Tai Chi skilled	10	women	50.5 (5.5)	not specified, 24 postures	6.3 (0.8)	60.4 (8.6)[1]	+1.13	+0.18	+2.07
			Tai Chi novice	10	women	53.6 (4.9)	–	0.8 (0.4)	49.3 (10.1)[1]			
Lan et al., 2004	cross-sectional	community dwelling non-smokers	Tai Chi	12	men	58.8 (7.9)	Yang, 108 postures	4.7 (2.3)	32.5 (4.9)	+1.83	+0.88	+2.79
			sedentary	12	men	59.9 (5.2)	–		24.3 (3.6)			

ES = Effect size; LBCI = lower bound confidence interval; UBCI = upper bound confidence interval; asterisk signifies matched on gender, age and body composition. Figures in parentheses indicate SD. ES is not significant if zero is included in the confidence interval.
[1]Estimated VO$_{2max}$.

Data Analyses

Calculation of Effect Sizes

The effect sizes (ESs) were calculated from the standardized mean differences using means and standard deviations reported for aerobic capacity (peak oxygen uptake). The standardized mean difference ES, also called d, is a scale-free measure that can contrast results for two groups, with continuous underlying distributions [10, 27]. ESs are important for power calculations when designing research studies, and help clinicians and researchers understand the magnitude and direction of a relationship [27, 28].

D-STAT software was used to calculate the ES and the 95% confidence intervals [29]. The ES for each study was weighted by the sample size and pooled variance. The postintervention mean peak oxygen uptake was used to contrast the experimental and control group in the experimental studies, as there was no significant difference in the baseline mean scores in these studies. The ES in the cross-sectional studies were derived from group contrasts between the Tai Chi and comparison groups. All relevant data derived from the studies were coded and entered into SPSS [26] for analysis.

Interpretation of ESs

ES guidelines from Cohen [27] are commonly used as a rule of thumb for interpreting ES results, with an ES of 0.20 considered a small effect, 0.50 a moderate effect and 0.80 a large effect [27]. In addition, a proportion of variance (η^2) between two groups can be calculated. Finally, interpretation of the ES can be expanded by transforming the ES into a percentile. The percentile is obtained by referring to a normal distribution table and identifying the area under the curve associated with the ES, referred to as the measure of nonoverlap (U_3) [27, 28]. U_3 is the percentage of the control distribution exceeded by the upper 50% of the treatment population. U_3 readily provides the clinician with information regarding the success or failure, of a treatment or intervention. For example, if the ES = 0.86, then 81% of the control group is below the average person in the treatment group.

ES Analyses Plan

Aerobic capacity is influenced by many factors including gender, age, exercise habits, weight, genetic factors and cardiovascular clinical status. Effects of Tai Chi exercise on aerobic capacity calculated in this meta-analysis included study design, gender, age, and type of comparison group (sedentary, other physical activity). For age, a cutpoint of 55 years was used, given that women are generally postmenopausal by that time, and patterns of chronic disease begin to develop at that age.

Results

Study Characteristics

A quality score was given for each of the studies included in this meta-analysis. Scores ranged from 21 to 30 (mean = 25.2, SD = 2.2) and no studies were excluded on the basis of their quality. In the experimental studies, the average length of the Tai Chi exercise intervention was 26 ± 19 weeks (range = 12–52 weeks), with a 20% attrition rate on average (range = 0–41%). In the cross-sectional studies, the number of years subjects practiced Tai Chi was 8 ± 2.7 years (range = 4.7–11.8 years). Study populations participating in these studies were mainly healthy, community-dwelling adults (71%), though several studies included those with a chronic disease (29%) such as coronary artery disease, chronic heart failure, hypertension and osteoarthritis. Peak oxygen uptake was mainly measured using cycle ergometers (78.9%), though treadmill testing was also reported (21.1%). The Yang style of Tai Chi was the principal style used (73.7%), followed by the Sun style (5.3%), while 21.1% of the studies did not specify the style of Tai Chi used.

There were a total of 322 Tai Chi subjects (182 women, 140 men) participating in these studies. They were on average 60.6 ± 8.9 years old (range = 35.5–71.5 years), with an average of 17 ± 8 Tai Chi subjects enrolled per study (range = 7–38 subjects/group). There were a total of 323 control/comparison subjects (183 women, 140 men). These subjects were similar in age (mean = 60.4 ± 9.4 years old, range = 30–73.5 years) and in the number of subjects per group enrolled in the studies (mean = 17 ± 7 subjects/group, range = 8–34 subjects/group).

Effects of Tai Chi on Aerobic Capacity

Effects of Tai Chi exercise on aerobic capacity calculated in this meta-analysis included study design, gender, age, and type of comparison group. The ES and the 95% confidence interval were calculated for each study, weighted by the sample size and pooled variance. The percent of variance between groups (η^2) and the measure of nonoverlap (U_3), were only calculated for effects found to be statistically significant (table 3).

The average ES for the experimental studies was small (ES = 0.38, CI = −0.10 to 0.85) and not statistically significant (fig. 2), which is in contrast to the cross-sectional studies where the average ES was large (ES = 1.33, CI = 0.91–1.75) (fig. 3). In the cross-sectional studies, approximately 31% ($\eta^2 = 0.31$) of the variance in aerobic capacity could be explained. Aerobic capacity for the average subject in a Tai Chi exercise group was higher than 91% of the subjects in the comparison groups, in the cross-sectional studies.

Gender-specific effects were calculated on studies reporting gender-specific results. The effect of Tai Chi on improving aerobic capacity in both women and men were large (1.09 and 0.86, respectively; table 3). Aerobic capacity for the average woman in a Tai Chi exercise group was higher than 86% of the women in the comparison groups. Aerobic capacity for the average man in a Tai Chi exercise group was higher than 81% of the men in the comparison groups.

16 Liu Y, Mimura K, Wang L, Ikuda K: Physiological benefits of 24-style Taijiquan exercise in middle-aged women. J Physiol Anthropol Appl Human Sci 2003;22:219–225.

17 Wang JS, Lan C, Chen SY, Wong MK: Tai Chi Chuan training is associated with enhanced endothelium-dependent dilation in skin vasculature of healthy older men. J Am Geriatr Soc 2002;50:1024–1030.

18 Brown DR, Wang Y, Ward A, Ebbeling CB, Fortlage L, Puleo E, et al: Chronic psychological effects of exercise and exercise plus cognitive strategies. Med Sci Sports Exerc 1995;27:765–775.

19 Lan C, Chen SY, Lai JS, Wong MK: The effect of Tai Chi on cardiorespiratory function in patients with coronary artery bypass surgery. Med Sci Sports Exerc 1999;31:634–638.

20 Lan C, Lai JS, Chen SY, Wong MK: 12-month Tai Chi training in the elderly: its effect on health fitness. Med Sci Sports Exerc 1998;30:345–351.

21 Young DR, Appel LJ, Jee S, Miller ER 3rd: The effects of aerobic exercise and T'ai Chi on blood pressure in older people: results of a randomized trial. J Am Geriatr Soc 1999;47:277–284.

22 Lai JS, Wong MK, Lan C, Chong CK, Lien IN: Cardiorespiratory responses of Tai Chi Chuan practitioners and sedentary subjects during cycle ergometry. J Formos Med Assoc 1993;92: 894–899.

23 Lan C, Lai JS, Wong MK, Yu ML: Cardiorespiratory function, flexibility, and body composition among geriatric Tai Chi Chuan practitioners. Arch Phys Med Rehabil 1996;77:612–616.

24 Schneider D, Leung R: Metabolic and cardiorespiratory responses to the performance of Wing Chun and T'ai Chi Chuan exercise. Int J Sports Med 1991;12:319–323.

25 Chan WW, Bartlett DJ: Effectiveness of Tai Chi as therapeutic exercise in improving balance and postural control. Phys Occup Ther Geri 2000;17:1–22.

26 Norusis MJ: SPSS 10.0: Guide to data analysis. Upper Saddle River, N.J.: Prentice Hall, 2000.

27 Cohen J: Statistical power analysis for the behavioral sciences, ed 2. Hillsdale N.J.: Lawerence Erlbaum Associates, 1988.

28 Lipsey MW, Wilson DB: Practical meta-analysis. Thousand Oaks, CA, Sage, 2001.

29 Johnson BT: D-STAT: Software for the meta-analytic review of research literature. Lawrence Erlbaum Associates, Inc., 1989.

30 Haskell WL. J.B: Wolffe Memorial Lecture. Health consequences of physical activity: understanding and challenges regarding dose-response. Med Sci Sports Exerc 1994;26:649–660.

Ruth E. Taylor-Piliae, PhD, R.N.
Assistant Professor
College of Nursing, The University of Arizona
1305 N. Martin, PO Box 210203
Tucson, AZ 85721-0203 (USA)
Tel. +1 520 626 4881, Fax +1 520 626 4062, E-Mail rtaylor@nursing.arizona.edu

Hong Y (ed): Tai Chi Chuan. State of the Art in International Research.
Med Sport Sci. Basel, Karger, 2008, vol 52, pp 54–63

....

Tai Chi Exercise in Improving Cardiorespiratory Capacity

Everard W. Thornton

School of Psychology, University of Liverpool, Liverpool, UK

Abstract

Introduction/Purpose: To evaluate evidence relating to effects of Tai Chi on cardio-vascular outcomes, with emphasis on randomised control designs. **Procedure:** Studies reviewed in 2004 were re-examined, together with more recent controlled trials of Tai Chi relating to cardiovascular outcome. The analysis provided comment on problems associated with randomised control design, including sources of bias in such trials. **Results:** With a single exception, data support reduction of *baseline* systolic/diastolic blood pressure (BP). While there may be positive bias in these studies, data are from diverse ethnic groups, different gender, age, and level of functional ability. There are no data relating to BP reactive change to subsequent stressors. Few studies consider potential mediating mechanisms through which Tai Chi may provide these benefits. **Implications:** Caution is advocated in using randomised controlled trials as the only effective type of study. Such designs are difficult to conduct and effective trials are more likely given a better understanding of the mediating mechanism(s) through which benefits may be derived. It is currently unclear how changes in BP are derived. Some data indicate a shift to increased vagal relative to sympathetic dominance and there may be other potential physiological mediators. No study has examined relationships between potential psychological gains such as self-efficacy and BP change, or individual differences in outcomes.

Copyright © 2008 S. Karger AG, Basel

There is considerable evidence to suggest Tai Chi enhances general well-being and possibly conveys health benefits. The documented outcomes are diverse and include general physical function such as mobility, strength and flexibility, balance, falls, fear of falling, improved mood and several dimensions of quality of life. Such improvements are documented using both self-report scales and objective measurement. However, much supportive data is based on pre-/post-testing of selected samples of participants and such a procedure may introduce positive bias, most obviously when the evidence is derived from current Tai Chi practitioners. Alternatively, a positive bias may be introduced because of significant numbers of dropouts, with only those for whom benefits are experienced completing post-exercise testing. Further positive bias may exist because much of the evidence is based on elderly cohorts, partly because the features of low velocity, low impact and low technical nature of the exercise make Tai Chi especially suitable for the elderly. Nevertheless, the elderly are often inactive and take little exercise and, as a consequence, such 'floor' effects mean that any 'activity' is likely to enhance well-being. Bias becomes greater when the population sampled has a problem in the area relevant to the selected dependent measure. In essence, positive outcomes are contaminated by a combination of a floor effect and regression to the mean. If, for example, a population with hypertension is selected, then any second measurement is likely to move in a normotensive direction even without an underlying change in the cardiovascular function. The same arguments apply for evaluation of Tai Chi based on selection of participants with poor balance. While this may be an appropriate group to target in an intervention, any second test may show improvement. Adaptation to the test procedures and the well-established 'Hawthorne Effect' wherein any intervention applied as a novel independent variable is likely to result in improved performance, are additional forms of bias in favour of likely beneficial outcomes from Tai Chi.

This analysis indicates that the quality of much of this evidence in support of Tai Chi may be weak with few randomised controlled trials (RCTs), the 'accepted' standard for scientific support. Two reviews of the outcomes following Tai Chi in RCTs indicate just how few randomised controlled studies had been undertaken prior to 2004. Verhagen et al. [1] restricted their sampling to those aged 50 years or more, and reported only nine articles that filled the basic criteria for an RCT design. Three of these were actually from the same (FICSIT) trial; five of these were related to cardiovascular function, and of the nine only five had more than 25 participants. The second review by Wang et al. [2] examined 743 citations concerning Tai Chi and chronic health conditions from 1966 to 2002 and excluded 679 on the basis that they provided poor or absent data. Of the remaining 64, only 9 could be classified as RCTs, with 23 non-randomised studies and 15 observational studies. Only 2 of the RCTs related to cardiovascular function. Unsurprisingly, both reviews commented that the 'scientific' evidence in support of benefits from Tai Chi is limited, a conclusion supported in a more recent review that adds little analysis but does importantly comment on the need for studies in younger age cohorts and longer-term follow-up [3]. The comment challenges whether expectations for Tai Chi should be directed toward healthy aging rather than more immediate clinical benefits. If the former, then the absence of follow-up of over the long-term in most studies cited in these reviews is a further limitation.

The need to support potential benefits from Tai Chi, the clinical imperative, is most evident in studies that have invoked Tai Chi as an exercise for enhancing outcomes for diverse groups of cardiovascular patients, including those with hypertension [4, 5] heart failure [6], cardiac infarction [7] and stroke [8], or following coronary artery bypass surgery [9]. In support of these interventions, others have examined dependent measures related to enhanced 'risk' for cardiovascular events in non-patient participants. These include blood pressure (BP) [10, 11], autonomic balance [12, 13] and cholesterol/lipid profile [4, 5].

Several studies, most notably the contributions from Lan et al. [9, 14], Taylor Piliae et al. [11] and Taylor Piliae and Froelicher [15], with diverse forms of Tai Chi undertaken in different continents with different ethnic populations and gender, indicate that Tai Chi invokes a demand equal to 50–65% of VO_{2max} (55–65% of heart rate reserve). These changes in aerobic capacity have been documented using both direct and estimated methods with similar values in young, middle-aged and older participants [14]. These studies are important because they provide evidence that Tai Chi is an aerobic exercise of moderate intensity, with the majority suggesting an intensity of approximately 4 METS (metabolic equivalents – range 1.5–6 METS). These data on aerobic capacity provide indirect support for Tai Chi in cardiovascular disease since a larger literature has indicated the benefits of other forms of aerobic exercise for cardiovascular health outcomes over the lifespan [16].

Before considering the outcome from such RCTs, including those published since 2004, it is important to reflect both on the small number of studies and the inherent problems in effecting such studies. Firstly, it is impossible within the context of 'informed consent' to effect 'blinded' trials with respect to participants, especially clinical populations. Secondly, while control groups may be comprised to minimise variables such as attention and/or demand characteristics it is not possible to be sure these factors are eliminated by 'control' procedures since groups can be matched only in terms of limited parameters, such as number of sessions and social context. Thirdly, while double-blind trials have become the accepted scientific standard for acute medical interventions, including drug trials, it is less sensible to ask for similar standards for behavioural or psychological interventions, and the latter may indeed apply as the salient mediator of improvements in cardiovascular function for Tai Chi. As an example, participants cannot be 'blinded' with respect to intervention. Fourthly, it may be difficult to conceal and/or withdraw benefits from control groups and so control conditions may become 'contaminated'.

A useful analysis of non-experimental, quasi-experimental and experimental studies designed to demonstrate beneficial psychological effects of exercise [17] indicates positive features for improved experimental design and such analysis is appropriate for the design of effective studies to investigate potential benefits of Tai Chi. In recognising the benefits of effective experimental designs and reflecting on the problems of RCTs with respect to clinical outcomes, improved studies can be effected in applied research. However, the scientific and clinical imperative provides a danger in the evaluation of such interventions. Even when there is substantial phenomenological, cross-sectional and correlative data, negative outcomes from such trials may be interpreted as indicating that the variable in question, here Tai Chi, is not effective in providing change for the dependent variable of concern: Do we throw out the baby with the bathwater? Two examples with respect to cardiovascular patients and health outcome that have direct implications for the effectiveness of Tai Chi may be cited since they relate to psychosocial mediators associated with benefits from Tai Chi and each have been directly related to increased sympathetic activity and increased BP. First, depression and treatment for depression: while depression in patients after myocardial infarction is associated with poor outcome [18], treatment for depression that does improve depression has not provided a reduction in secondary episodes [19]. The second example invokes 'the reactivity hypothesis' that suggests stress is associated with sympathetic hyper-reactivity and that sympathetic dysfunction is associated with coronary status. Despite support for the reactivity hypothesis in acute studies documenting cardiovascular changes during a stressor, the more specific relationship between acute vascular changes to stressors and the development of hypertension remains controversial [20].

The alternative strategy is to continue attempts to identify/specify underlying causal mechanisms since the case for a 'beneficial factor' for good health is strengthened if such mediators are identified. The concentration on an established risk factor for cardiovascular disease, BP as *the* exclusive mediating mechanism may be misplaced. The beneficial outcomes for cardiovascular patients related to BP may be derived from improved vagal autonomic dominance or decreased immunological markers. Psychological variables such as improved mood state, more specifically reduced anxiety and/or depression, may be more important mediators and these in turn may be provided through an increase in personal self-efficacy. While the primary objective may be improved clinical outcomes, empirical investigation may be better directed to examination of these more proximal mediating variables. Examples of positive contributions are those that have examined both psychological mediators of the benefits of Tai Chi such as self-efficacy [21] and physiological mediators such as autonomic balance [22], sympathetic reactivity [23] and serum B-natriuretic peptide [6]. Such studies enable us to better understand the mechanisms through which Tai Chi conveys any clinical benefits. The mediation may be indirect and interactions may be important. For example, there may be a linear causal sequence such that self-efficacy may decrease negative mood, improve social interaction, decrease stress, thereby changing sympathetic dominance and BP. However, it is possible that the links in this sequential chain may be inverted in direction at certain points, or be more complex and/or non-linear. An example of the value of a focus on mediation is for falls, given evidence from RCTs that reduction in falls and injury following Tai Chi is equivocal, especially for community samples where baseline incidence rate may be low. In contrast to falls per se, the evidence for improved balance and muscle strength, potential mediators for falls, is much stronger. Empirical study of these variables is recommended, especially as evidence suggests that participants are more likely to be recruited and retained for a programme of balance than for falls per se, so reducing selection bias. While redirection of empirical study to such mediators of clinical end points is warranted, they still need to be carefully chosen and plausible ones evaluated. For example, tests of dynamic balance more closely relate to falls than static balance tests. Specifically in relation to cardiovascular function; while improved lipid profile may be a plausible mediator given extensive evidence that aerobic exercise in general has been shown to improve lipid profiles, studies of Tai Chi have not consistently provided such an outcome [4].

While there is selection bias in many studies and RCTs, the evidence does indicate that Tai Chi provides aerobic/cardiorespiratory benefit. Several of the studies cited indicate increases in VO_{2max} of 16–20% over 1 year following participation in Tai Chi, although a recent meta-analysis suggests the effects may be smaller [15]. The magnitude of the changes documented undoubtedly relates to the specific form of Tai Chi, the frequency and duration of the exercise and the duration over which change is assessed. Indeed, it is these diverse variables that require decisions for an RCT with respect to both the details of the Tai Chi programme and the duration of follow-up. The debate relates to both our expectancy for benefits from Tai Chi and the wider evidence relating to exercise and health. For the former, it is the debate about 'good aging' versus interventions for patients – treatment or prevention. For the latter, it is whether benefits relate to activity or physical fitness. Debates about levels of aerobic exercise that convey benefits for cardiovascular disease have oscillated between emphasis on vigorous aerobic exercise to overcoming a sedentary lifestyle. While there is much evidence to suggest that within limits 'more is better', benefits are apparent only if levels are ≥ 3 METS or 50% VO_{2max}, a threshold close to that of Tai Chi and how intensely it is performed. However, it has been argued that intensity is irrelevant and that it is *cumulative activity* that determines benefits. This begs the question as to what participants are doing at times other than the formal Tai Chi intervention programme during any RCT – a variable that has not been documented to date, and one unlikely in long-term follow-up. What has been established in favour of low-intensity exercise is improved adherence across participants as a whole, and long-term benefits with respect to health and aging accrue only with maintained practice. Personality variables, including a sense of control, may also be associated with both adherence and more general levels of activity. Such measures have not been incorporated into studies of the outcomes from Tai Chi interventions despite the fact that variables such as neuroticism are known to be associated with autonomic reactivity and personality types, such as the type D personality, are predictors of both the incidence and the outcomes of cardiovascular conditions. The failure to identify and document such powerful moderator variables is almost certain to influence outcomes from an RCT. Tai Chi may not benefit all and examination of such moderators will lead to better targeting and possibly more positive findings in RCTs. Despite these caveats and given aerobic gains from Tai Chi, the inferential case for health benefits is good – there is substantial evidence that diverse forms of exercise of low or moderate intensity convey substantial health benefits [24].

While advocating the merits of studies that have attempted to better understand potential mediators for beneficial effects of Tai Chi, with recent encouraging studies, there has also been an increase in improved controlled trials assessing cardiovascular benefits since the two excellent reviews of 2004 [1, 2]. Not all of these studies have randomised participants to group but, in quasi-experimental designs, they have attempted a matched control design. Several of these studies have been cited already in this commentary; other studies that have provided non-experimental designs over this period are not reviewed. The studies are listed in table 1. Two studies [12, 23] were directed primarily to examining mediators of benefits from Tai Chi and assessed between-group outcomes only acutely during and immediately after Tai Chi exercise. The follow-up period for the remaining studies was extended and ranged from 6 weeks to 12 months, although only 2 recent studies provided 1-year outcomes [25, 26], with the large majority assessing outcomes after 12 weeks. The most frequent dependent measures were *baseline* change in systolic and diastolic BP (SDP, DBP) and all but one study [26] provided reductions in SBP after only 12 weeks despite the very different ages and nature of the participants. For example, in our study [10] the decrease of approximately 9 mm Hg was similar to that provided in the earliest study. The decreases in the younger, non-clinical population were rather larger than the 5 mm Hg at 3 months reported in the extended study of Wolf et al. [25] with a frail elderly population where the intensity of exercise is likely to have been low. Unsurprisingly, given the present analysis, the largest reductions reported are for participants in two studies with participants with initial high BP [4, 5] and for whom decreases of 19 and 15 mm Hg, respectively, were reported. The one study reporting no beneficial change in BP also reported absence of change in several other non-cardiovascular variables [26]. Nevertheless, this

Table 1. Experimental studies of effects of Tai Chi on cardiovascular responses from 2003

Authors	Age and sample	Country	Population[1]	Design	Duration	Outcome[2]
Tsai et al. [4]	51 years (mean); borderline hypertensives; n = 78	Taiwan	Chinese	RCT	12 weeks	SBP, DBP and serum cholesterol decreased; HDL increased
Thornton et al. [10][3]	33–55 years; healthy women; n = 34	Hong Kong	Chinese	RCT	12 weeks	SBP and DBP decreased
Yeh et al. [6][3]	64 years (mean); heart failure patients; n = 30	USA	Caucasian	RCT	12 weeks	BP not reported; decreased serum B natriuretic peptide
Lee [5]	hypertensive elderly; n = 28	Korea	Korean	Non-matched controls	6 weeks	SBP and DBP decreased; cholesterol unchanged; cortisol unchanged
Lu and Kuo [12]	TCC practitioners, healthy elderly; n = 40	Taiwan	Chinese	TCC group, non-matched controls	During TC and to 60 min after exercise	HRV lower in practitioners; enhanced vagal balance in both groups after exercise
Taylor-Piliae et al. [11]	>45 years; community sample; at risk CVD	USA	Chinese	Quasi-experimental	12 weeks	SBP and DBP decreased; aerobic power (indirect) increased
Wolf et al.[25][3]	70–97 years; frail, independent residential centres	USA	Caucasian	RCT	12 months	SBP and HR decreased; DBP no difference
Motivala et al. [23]	60–85 years; n = 8	USA	Caucasian	TCC group; non-matched controls	Acute changes 10 min before and after exercise	Pre-ejection period decrease: decreased sympathetic effect; no group difference in BP

Study	Sample	Location	Ethnicity[1]	Design	Duration	Comments[2]
Thomas et al. [26][3]	65–74 years; healthy; n = 207	Hong Kong	Chinese	RCT × 3 groups: TC, resistance exercise, control	12 months	No change in BP; no change in lipids/cholesterol *only* resistance group increased insulin sensitivity
Audette et al. [13][3]	71 years (mean); women only; sedentary	USA	Caucasian	RCT (partly) ×3 groups: TC, walking, control	12 weeks	BP changes not reported; HRV changes indicating increased vagal and decreased sympathetic function; aerobic power (indirect) increased

TC = Tai Chi; TCC = Tai Chi Chuan; HR = heart rate; HRV = heart rate variability.

[1]Ethnicity relates to the majority of the sample.

[2]Comments here relate to between-group effects where relevant rather than pre- to post-change in the dependent variable.

[3]Studies also document functional/behavioural dependent variables.

study was well designed and the negative outcome, especially for a Chinese population where cultural support exists, should not be lightly dismissed. The 'explanation' cited by the authors, specifically the possible decrease in alternative forms of activity in their participants, has been empirically documented in other studies when individuals undertake a formal exercise programme. This emphasises the need to assess wider diary information from participants in an RCT that may influence dependent measures, including activity and diet.

Not one of the 10 trials cited in table 1 took the opportunity to correlate change in the dependent measure of interest with any potential mediator. Obvious possibilities are correlates between self-efficacy or mood, BP change and aerobic gain. More positively, however, several studies have assessed alternative physiological variables that relate to cardiovascular pathology [4–6, 12, 23, 26], supporting an awareness of the need to examine alternative mediators to that of BP. Unfortunately, no study has examined a change in BP *reactivity to challenge* following Tai Chi exercise, or the return to baseline following such challenge.

In conclusion, there have been an increasing number of controlled trials that indicate benefits from Tai Chi for cardiovascular function, although not without exception. There may be a positive bias in the literature for publication of studies towards those reporting positive outcomes. It is recommended that future studies incorporate within participant correlation analyses within experimental designs to better identify mediator variables and to delineate participants for whom this form of exercise conveys benefits. It is also important to consider the possibility that benefits for different individual are dependent on different mediators. If we are to have better RCTs, it is necessary to have a more clear understanding of the mechanisms through which changes in cardiovascular variables are effected. RCTs are important but they are not the only way forward and the need may not be for simply bigger and better trials but trials that either target populations or incorporate moderator variables/plausible mediators that then provide a better understanding of the outcomes from such trials.

References

1   Verhagen AP, Immink K, Van Der Meulen A, Bierma-Zeinstra SMA: The efficacy of Tai Chi Chuan in older adults: a systematic review. Family Prac 2004;21:107–113.
2   Wang C, Collet JP, Lau J: The effect of Tai Chi on health outcomes in patients with chronic conditions. Arch Intern Med 2004;164:493–501.
3   Kuramoto AM: Therapeutic benefits of Tai Chi exercise: a research review. WMJ 2006;105:42–46.
4   Tsai JC, Wang WH, Chan P, Lin LJ, Wang CH, Tomlinson B, Hsieh MH, Yang HU, Liu JC: The beneficial effects of Tai Chi Chuan on blood pressure and lipid profile and anxiety status in a randomised controlled design. J Alt Compl Med 2003;9:747–754.
5   Lee EN: The effects of tai chi exercise program on blood pressure, total cholesterol and cortisol level in patients with hypertension. Taehan Kanho Chi 2004;34:829–837.

6   Yeh GY, Wood MJ, Lorell BH, Stevenson LW, Elsenberg DM, Wayne PM, Goldberger AL, Davis RB, Phillips RS: Effects of tai chi mind-body therapy on functional status and exercise capacity inpatients with chronic heart failure: a randomised control trial. Am J Med 2004;117:541–548.

7   Channer KS, Barrow D, Osborne M, Ives G: Changes in hemodynamic parameters following Tai Chi Chuan and aerobic exercise in patients recovering from myocardial infarction. Post Med J 1996;72:349–351.

8   Hart J, Kanner H, Gilboa-Mayo R, Haroeh-Peer O, Rozenthul-Sorokin N, Eldar R: Tai Chi Chuan practice in community dwelling persons after stroke. Int J Rehab Res 2004;27:303–304.

9   Lan C, Chen SY, Lai JS, Wong MK: The effect of tai chi on cardiorespiratory function in patients with coronary artery bypass surgery. Med Sci Sports Exerc 1999;31:634–638.

10 Thornton EW, Sykes KS, Tang WK: Health benefits of Tai Chi exercise: improved balance and blood pressure in middle-aged women. Hlth Promot Int 2004;19:33–38.

11 Taylor-Piliae RE, Haskell WL, Froelicher ES: Hemodynamic responses to community-based Tai Chi exercise in ethnic Chinese adults with cardiovascular disease risk factors. Eur J Cardiovasc Nurs 2006;5:165–174.

12 Lu WA, Kuo CD: The effect of Tai Chi Chuan on the autonomic nervous modulation in older persons. Med Sci Sports Exerc 2003;12:1972–1976.

13 Audette JF, Jin YS, Newcomer R, Stein L, Ducan G, Frontera WR: Tai Chi versus brisk walking in elderly women. Age Ageing 2006;35:388–393.

14 Lan C, Chen SY, Lai JS: Relative exercise intensity of Tai Chi Chuan is similar in different ages and gender. Am J Chin Med 2004;32:151–160.

15 Taylor-Piliae RE, Froelicher ES: Effectiveness of Tai Chi exercise in improving aerobic capacity: a meta-analysis. J Cardiovsc Nurs 2004;19:48–57.

16 Lee IM, Paffenbarger RS: Associations of light, moderate, and vigorous intensity physical activity with longevity. Am J Epidemiol 2000;151:293–299.

17 Folkins CH, Sime WE: Physical fitness training and mental health. Am Psychol 1981;36:373–389.

18 Frasure-Smith N, Lesperance F, Talajic M: Depression and 18-month prognosis after myocardial infarction. Circulation 1995;91:999–1005.

19 Glassman AH, O'Connor CM, Califf RM, Swedberg K, Schwartz P, Bigger JT, et al: Sertraline treatment of major depression in patients with acute MI or unstable angina. JAMA 2002;288: 701–709.

20 Carroll D, Davey Smith G, Sheffield D, Shipley MJ, Marmot MG: Pressor reactions to psychological stress and prediction of future blood pressure: data from the Whitehall II study. Br Med J 1995;310:771–776.

21 Li F, McAuley E, Harmer P, Ducan TE, Chaumeton NR: Tai Chi enhances self-efficacy and exercise behavior in older adults. J Aging Phys Activity 2001;9:161–171.

22 Lu WA, Kuo CD: The effect of Tai Chi Chuan on the autonomic nervous modulation in older persons. Med Sci Sports Exerc 2003;35:1972–1976.

23 Motivala SJ, Sollers J, Thayer J, Irwin MR: Tai Chi Chi acutely decreases sympathetic nervous system reactivity in older adults. J Gerontol Med Sci 2006;61A:1177–1180.

24 Press V, Freestone I, George CF: Physical activity: the evidence of benefit in the prevention of coronary heart disease. Q J Med 2003;96:245–251.

25 Wolf SL, O'Grady M, Easley KA, Ying G, Kressig RW, Kutner M: The influence of intense Tai Chi training on physical performance and hemodynamic outcomes in transitionally frail, older adults. J Gerontol Med Sci 2006;61A:184–189.

26 Thomas GN, Hong AWL, Tomlinson B, Lau E, Lamb CWK, Sanderson JE: Effects of Tai Chi and resistance training on cardiovascular risk factors in elderly Chinese subjects: a 12-month longitudinal, randomized, controlled intervention study. Clin Endocrinol 2005;63:663–669.

Everard W. Thornton, PhD
School of Psychology, University of Liverpool
Liverpool L69 7ZA (UK)
Tel. +44 151 794 2948, Fax +44 151 794 6937, E-Mail ewt1@liverpool.ac.uk

Hong Y (ed): Tai Chi Chuan. State of the Art in International Research.
Med Sport Sci. Basel, Karger, 2008, vol 52, pp 64–76

• •

Effects of a Traditional Taiji/Qigong Curriculum on Older Adults' Immune Response to Influenza Vaccine

Yang Yang[a,c], Jay Verkuilen[b], Karl S. Rosengren[a,b], Rachel A. Mariani[a], Michael Reed[a,c], Scott A. Grubisich[c], Jeffrey A. Woods[a], Bob Schlagal[c]

Departments of [a]Kinesiology and Community Health and [b]Psychology, University of Illinois at Urbana-Champaign, Urbana-Champaign, Ill., and [c]Center for Taiji Studies, Champaign, Ill., USA

Abstract

Previous studies have suggested that Taiji (T'ai Chi) practice may improve immune function. The current study examined whether 5 months of moderate traditional Taiji and Qigong (TQ) practice could improve the immune response to influenza vaccine in older adults. Fifty older adults participated in this study. Baseline pre-vaccine blood samples were collected. Subjects received the 2003–2004 influenza vaccine during the 1st week of the intervention. Post-vaccine blood samples were collected 3, 6 and 20 weeks after intervention for analysis of anti-influenza hemagglutination inhibition titers. Findings indicated a significant increase in the magnitude and duration of the antibody response to influenza vaccine in TQ participants when compared to controls. There was a significant between-group difference at 3 and 20 weeks after vaccine, and at 20 weeks the TQ group had significantly higher titers compared to the pre-vaccine time point, whereas the controls did not. A higher percentage of TQ subjects also responded to the influenza A strains with a protective antibody response, but differences between groups were not statistically significant. Traditional TQ practice improves the antibody response to influenza vaccine in older adults, but further study is needed to determine whether the enhanced response is sufficient to provide definitive protection from influenza infection.

Copyright © 2008 S. Karger AG, Basel

The health of older adults is a topic of increasing concern amid aging populations in North America and elsewhere in the world. In particular, influenza is a topic of annual concern for this age group. Each year, the influenza virus is responsible for an estimated 36,000 deaths and up to 150,000 hospitalizations in the United States [1]. Persons above 65 years of age are at increased risk of serious illness and death, especially those with chronic diseases [1–3]. The most effective means of influenza virus prevention is administration of the influenza vaccine. Although the vaccine is usually effective at preventing serious illness and death in young adults, a large percentage of older adults do not typically generate protective levels of antibodies to the flu vaccine [4, 5]. These realities have led to research aimed at identifying factors that can lessen influenza incidence and severity and/or improve influenza vaccine efficacy.

In recent years, there has been an expanding interest in alternative and complementary therapies, although few studies have examined the impact of holistic or behavioral interventions on immune function. One popular, yet understudied therapy is Taiji (T'ai Chi), a fusion of martial arts with Daoist philosophy and traditional Chinese medicine [6]. Many studies on older adults report that Taiji improves quality of life, flexibility, strength, cardiovascular function, pain, balance, and kinesthetic sense [7–9]. The use of Taiji as a behavioral intervention in older adults is particularly attractive due to age-related loss of function and problems with even moderate intensity exercise interventions. One recent study also found that a Westernized form of Taiji led to a 50% improvement in the immune response to varicella zoster virus (the shingles virus) in a small group of healthy older adults [10]. These results suggest that Taiji may alter immunity in the elderly. The purpose of this study was to determine whether traditional Taiji and Qigong practice may improve the antibody response to influenza vaccine in sedentary older adults.

A Traditional Taiji Curriculum

Most studies of the effects of Taiji on various aspects of health and well-being have used the practice of Taiji form alone as their intervention. While the slow movement that is most commonly recognized as Taiji is certainly a cornerstone of Taijiquan training, it is only one aspect of the art. Through the centuries, three forms of Taiji practice have evolved to form an efficient and comprehensive curriculum:
  – Qigong: Principally forms of sitting and standing meditation
  – Taiji form: Mainly slow movement practice
  – Push-hands: Two-person balance, strength, and reaction training

Each of these forms of practice is interrelated and synergistic – each exercise builds upon skills developed from the others. Further, it is a truism of Taiji training that the combined effects of correct practice of all exercises are greater than practice of individual exercises. In this study we elected to use two of the traditional practices – form and Qigong – but for practical purposes, not the

---

third[1]. Broadening the curriculum to include both form and Qigong practice, not only captures more of the tradition, but also appears to deepen the health benefits. In a recent study at the University of Illinois, the Taiji/Qigong effect was significant for balance and lower body strength *2 months* after beginning an intervention [Yang et al., unpubl. data]. The seven-movement choreographed Taiji form taught during the intervention was not memorized by the participants until the end of the 4th month; therefore, much of the credit for the rapid improvement in strength and balance must be attributed to the sitting and standing meditation component of the intervention curriculum. Therefore, both were included in this study.

Sitting and Standing Qigong Meditation

Standing Qigong meditation is literally translated from the Chinese as 'standing pole' or 'standing post' exercise and is the basis for Taiji movement. In fact, the Taiji form movement is often referred to as 'moving pole', highlighting the fact that Taiji movement is rooted in the practice of standing meditation. Both the classical literature of Taijiquan and the oral tradition of the internal martial arts repeatedly emphasize that standing training is integral to Taiji movement.

Sitting and standing meditation are related exercises but yield different benefits. Both are 'mind/body' integrative exercises of the nervous system and both strengthen core musculature – upon which the mechanics of Taiji movement fundamentally rely. However, in general, sitting meditation is directed relatively more toward training the former (central nervous system) and standing to the latter (core strength). The standing and sitting meditation exercises are so crucial to efficient Taiji practice that it is precisely these exercises that were omitted from public teaching when the goal was to preserve the 'secret' of the art within a small, select group of family members or disciples. These practices are now an 'open secret', but little information has yet been disseminated as to *why* they are important, and almost none of the current Taiji research mentions them.

---

[1]Although push-hands is a foundational aspect of Taiji practice and is essential to realize the maximum possible benefits of practice, correct practice requires a foundation of skill developed through standing and sitting meditation and form practice. It is the first author's conclusion that push-hands can be practiced and enjoyed by older adults, but that there is little purpose in introducing this practice at the beginning stages of an intervention. Further information concerning the purpose and interrelated nature of the sitting and standing meditation, form, and push-hands exercises, including hypothesized mechanisms, is detailed in Yang and Grubisich [6].

Choreographed Form Movement

Over the last several hundred years, varied expressions or styles of Taiji have developed.

Although these different forms of Taiji vary in outward appearance, the principles of the movements remain the same. Understanding the mechanics of movement – as opposed to memorizing a specific choreography – is what is important in understanding Taiji movement. Once the essential mechanics are understood, any movement can be done as Taiji movement. Hence the 'style' or outward appearance of choreography is ultimately unimportant, but the principles of practice and mechanics of movement are essential and define 'Taiji movement'.

For beginning practitioners in general and older adults in particular, we developed and observed the following guidelines to ensure accessibility of our Taiji form to older adults while retaining the appropriate character of Taiji exercise:

– Form movements should not be overly complicated. While truly complex movements were omitted, some demanding postures, such as kicking motions requiring single leg stance or backwards walking motions, were retained to challenge healthy participants of any age.

– Range of motion should be as large as comfortably allowed. Beginners should gradually increase the range of motion of form movements to improve physical capabilities. Within the comfortable limit of ability, each practitioner should approach the maximum comfortable limits of waist turning and weight shifting during form practice. Doing so increases range of motion around the body joints while increasing the comfortable range of motion within the base of support, effectively increasing the radius about which one can maintain balance. (Once a person understands and can do a movement, however, it can be performed in any radius, big or small – there is no difference in the mechanics of how the movement is generated.) Therefore large movements were emphasized in our Taiji choreography.

– Varied directional movements should be included in the choreography. A wide variety of directional movement was used to challenge healthy practitioners of any age. Simply repeating the same or similar movements along a single directional line yields limited benefit in mind/body connection.

– Protect the knees. Postures and movements that are potentially injurious to the knees were avoided. According to Taiji principles, the knees should be slightly bent. However, beginning students of any age should not be encouraged to practice in lower postures. Besides violating basic Taiji principles, lower stances increase the risk of injury to the knees. Similarly, correct footwork must be employed so that the knees are not stressed during form movement. Postures and footwork should always be relaxed and natural – this requires constant stance adjustment during form practice.

Again, these differences in the complexity of movement and range of motion are applicable to and desirable for beginners of any age, and are described here as a variable subset of the general principles of Taiji practice and mechanics of Taiji movement.

Materials and Methods

Subjects

We recruited 41 subjects from a larger study examining sensory and strategic mechanisms of balance improvement afforded by a combined Taiji and Qigong (TQ) program for older adults [Yang, et al., unpubl. data]. Twenty-seven of those recruited had been assigned to the TQ intervention versus only 14 in the wait-list control (CON). Because of the large difference in subject number between groups, we recruited an additional 9 CON subjects using the same inclusion and exclusion criteria as the larger study for a final distribution of 27 and 23 in the TQ and CON groups, respectively. In this substudy, subjects were excluded if they were taking medications that altered immune responsiveness (e.g. corticosteroids or cancer therapies), or had conditions associated with immune dysfunction (e.g. severe autoimmune disorders or arthritis), neurological disorders, or had cognitive deficits as assessed by the Pfeiffer exam [11]. All subjects completed informed consent forms approved by the University Institutional Review Board. Each subject filled out a detailed medical history providing information about diagnosed diseases, medication use, general health problems, alcohol intake, smoking status and exercise participation. Each participant also completed the Pittsburgh Sleep Quality Index [12] to evaluate sleep quality. With respect to this substudy, 3 subjects dropped out of the Taiji intervention, one each at 5, 8 and 16 weeks. We were able to obtain post-vaccination blood samples from all of these subjects and included them in an intent-to-treat analysis.

Research Design and Intervention

The TQ group participated in three 1-hour classes per week for 20 weeks. The control group was asked to continue routine activities for the 20 weeks. Each 1-hour class consisted of equal parts of Qigong and Taiji form practice. The form consisted of 7 movements distilled from the Chen Style Essential 48 movement form. The seven movements selected focused on fundamental mobility skills: weight shifting to both sides (stepping and pivoting forward, backwards, sideways and diagonally), range of motion and coordination. They were also selected for their adaptability and accessibility. The forms were broken down into components that could be taught and practiced separately and then gradually connected by transitions until, by the 4th month, they could be performed continuously as a complete routine. The Qigong practice consisted of sitting and standing meditation. Students began with short periods of sitting. Standing was added in week 2 and times were gradually increased for both, until by the beginning of the 13th week participants were performing one 10-min sitting and two 10-min standing meditations in each 1-hour class. This combination of equal parts form and Qigong reflects the traditional Chinese training curriculum. The written and oral tradition of Chinese internal arts is clear on the primacy of standing and sitting meditation in nurturing complete and efficient development of Taiji's many benefits.

Pre-vaccine blood sampling and influenza vaccination occurred during the first week of the intervention. All subjects were vaccinated with a commercially available 2003–2004 influenza vaccine (Fluzone, Aventis-Pasteur, Swiftwater, Pa., USA) containing 15 μg of hemagglutinin from H1N1 (New Caledonia/20/99), H3N2 (Panama/2007/99), and B (Hong Kong/1434/2002) strains of the virus. Blood samples were taken 3, 6 and 20 weeks after the vaccination with the 20-week time point corresponding to the end of the intervention for this substudy. Serum samples were stored frozen at −80°C for later analysis.

Antibody Titer Analysis

Once all samples were collected, they were shipped frozen to a Center for Disease Control-affiliated reference laboratory (Hackensack Medical Center, Hackensack NJ) for blinded analysis of anti-influenza antibody titer by hemagglutination inhibition (HI) assay. Serial two-fold dilutions (e.g. 10–10,240) of participant sera were subject to HI assay performed using standard microtiter techniques, which included controls for nonspecific HI. The appropriate A and B test antigens for HI were obtained as egg allantoic fluid (WHO Collaborating Center for Influenza, Center for Disease Control, Atlanta, Ga., USA). All samples from a single subject were run in the same assay. In addition to raw antibody titer, we determined influenza vaccine efficacy as the percentage of subjects that responded to the vaccine with an antibody titer >40 HI (at any time point after vaccination), which is considered a titer sufficient to protect people from influenza infection [13].

Statistics

Student's t tests and χ^2 tests were performed to compare treatment groups on descriptive variables and χ^2 was used to explore differences in the percentage of subjects achieving protective HI responses. In order to assess the magnitude of change in HI antibody titers over time, we used a generalized estimating equations model for gamma-distributed responses. Because the dependent variable here has a strong right skew, the gamma distribution is an appropriate model. The generalized estimating equation model is widely used for the analysis of longitudinal biometric data.

Because the subjects were extremely diverse in their responses, we employed a within-subjects analysis. Subjects with missing data at a single time point (n = 11) were included in intent-to-treat design. Due to low statistical power associated with the small sample size, we pooled the HI antibody responses from the three different influenza strains included in the vaccine. This pooling was done using the geometric mean, which is an appropriate method of aggregation for variables that have a multiplicative relationship.

No problems were observed during model fitting. Because the sample size is relatively small, we used clustered-by-subjects bootstrapping to compute standard errors. To examine the effect in a more interpretable way, we generated predicted values for each treatment group by week, along with 99.2% confidence intervals. 99.2% gives the Bonferroni adjustment for six time and group comparisons, corresponding to an overall α-level of 0.05.

Results

Table 1 contains descriptive baseline information regarding the 50 participants in the intent-to-treat sample. There were no statistically significant differences in gender, weight, height, or BMI between the two groups. There was a borderline significant age difference between the two groups, with the Taiji

Table 1. Baseline comparisons between control and Taiji groups

Variable	Control (n = 23)	Taiji (n = 27)	Statistic; p value
Males/Females	7/16	6/21	$\chi^2 = 0.44; 0.54$
Age, years	74.5 ± 1.6	79.5 ± 1.9	t = 2.0; p = 0.05
Weight, kg	71.4 ± 2.0	63.9 ± 3.0	t = 1.9; p = 0.06
Height, cm	165 ± 1.8	162 ± 1.7	t = 1.1; p = 0.28
BMI	26.2 ± 0.57	24.1 ± 1.0	t = 1.7; p = 0.09
Diagnosed illnesses	3.4 ± 0.5	3.2 ± 0.5	t = 0.36; p = 0.72
Medications	4.0 ± 0.5	3.6 ± 0.5	t = 0.60; p = 0.55
PSQI	4.7 ± 0.8	5.3 ± 0.6	t = 0.56; p = 0.58
Exercise, times/week	3.8 ± 0.5	3.9 ± 0.5	t = 0.20; p = 0.84
Vitamin supplements	18/23	25/27	$\chi^2 = 0.53; 0.47$
Alcohol intake, oz/week	2.8 ± 0.9	1.1 ± 0.3	t = 1.9; p = 0.06
Baseline H1N1[1]	3.99 ± 0.28 (0–5.32)	3.78 ± 0.39 (0–7.32)	t = 0.42; p = 0.67
Baseline H3N2[1]	6.74 ± 0.53 (4.32–13.32)	6.0 ± 0.45 (0–10.32)	t = 1.1; p = 0.28
Baseline B[1]	6.00 ± 0.39 (3.32–10.32)	5.48 ± 0.48 (0–10.32)	t = 0.80; p = 0.42

PSQI = Pittsburg Sleep Quality Index.
[1] Expressed as log2 titer.

participants about 5 years older on average than controls. The groups were also similar in that there was no difference in the number of medications they took or the number of diagnosed diseases they were afflicted with. Sleep quality as measured by the PSQI was similar as was the number of times they exercised (≥20 min enough to 'break a sweat') each week. Groups were also similar in their intake of vitamin supplements and alcohol (table 1).

As prior influenza vaccination or exposure can alter pre-vaccine antibody titer and the net response to the influenza vaccine, we compared pre-vaccine HI titers between the two treatment groups. Importantly, there were no significant differences in pre-vaccine antibody titers between the Taiji and control groups (table 1), suggesting similar vaccine or exposure histories. We queried subjects about whether they had received the previous years' influenza vaccine (which contained identical strains to the 2003–2004 vaccine). Unfortunately, as is often the case in the elderly, 1 TQ and 3 control subjects could not remember if they had or had not received the previous years' shot. However, there were no differences between groups in the number of subjects that reported having the previous years' influenza vaccination (12/20 and 13/26 for control and TQ subjects, respectively; $\chi^2 = 0.46; 0.56$).

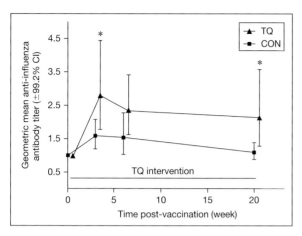

Fig. 1. Composite geometric mean HI antibody titers (±99.2% confidence interval) in CON (n = 23) and TQ (n = 27) subjects before and 3, 6 and 20 weeks after vaccination. Group comparisons revealed significantly elevated titers at 3 and 20 weeks after vaccination in the TQ when compared to the CON group (asterisks). With respect to time, both groups responded to the vaccine with significant elevations in titer at 3 and 6 weeks after vaccination. However, only the TQ group had significantly higher (when compared to pre-vaccination) titers at 20 weeks after vaccine.

The percentage attendance at the supervised TQ sessions over the course of the 20-week intervention was 80.5 ± 2.9% (range 23–96%). In questionnaires administered to the participants asking about TQ practice outside of the supervised sessions we found that the TQ group self-practiced the techniques an average of 2.8 ± 0.48 (range 0–7) times per week. The average length of a self-practice meditation session was 8.9 + 0.2 min (range 0–30 min).

Analysis of the HI titers can be found in figure 1. There was a statistically significant ($p < 0.05$) increase in predicted geometric mean antibody titer in the TQ when compared to the control group at the 3- and 20-week time points (note that the mean of the CON group falls outside the 99.2% CI). Compared to the pre-vaccine time point, vaccination of the CON group resulted in a statistically significant ($p < 0.05$) 58 and 54% increase in anti-influenza HI titer at 3 and 6 weeks post-vaccine, respectively. The anti-influenza titer at 20 weeks after vaccine (~10% increase) was not significantly different from the pre-vaccine time. This is in contrast to the statistically significant ($p < 0.05$) 173, 130, and 109% increases relative to pre-vaccine at 3, 6, and 20 weeks after vaccination, respectively, in the TQ group (fig. 1). We found no significant correlations between attendance or self-reported self-practice and maximal post-vaccination antibody responses ($r = 0.01$–0.3, $p > 0.05$); however, our sample size is quite

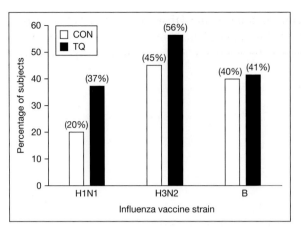

Fig. 2. Percentage of subjects that responded to the 2003–2004 influenza vaccine with a protective (e.g. ≥40 HI) response. Despite higher percentages in the Taiji group for the influenza A strains, χ^2 analysis revealed no statistically significant differences between groups in the percentage of study participants responding with protective responses (p = 0.21, 0.47, and 0.96 for H1N1, H3N2 and B strains, respectively).

low for an analysis of this type. Moreover, attendance at the sessions was relatively homogenous among the participants. Only one subject (23% attendance rate) was below 65%, with the majority of participants attending >80% of the supervised sessions.

Another way to examine influenza vaccine efficacy is to determine the percentage of people who developed a protective response (e.g. ≥40 HI) after vaccination [14]. As can be seen in figure 2, while more Taiji participants had a protective (e.g. ≥40 HI in response to the vaccine) titer response, particularly for the influenza A strains, this was not statistically significant via χ^2 analysis (p = 0.21, 0.47, and 0.96 for H1N1, H3N2 and B strains, respectively).

Discussion

This is the first study to examine the influence of a Taiji intervention on the response to influenza vaccine in older adults. Influenza is a major problem for this population because of age-related immunodysregulation that contributes to increased susceptibility, longer recovery, and failure to become adequately immunized when given the influenza vaccine [13]. Many strategies have been employed to improve influenza vaccine efficacy in the elderly. In this study, we found that 5 months of an easily performed behavioral Taiji and Qigong intervention could improve the magnitude and duration of the HI anti-influenza antibody titer response in a small cohort of older adults. Unfortunately, while there was a statistically significant increase in the amount of anti-influenza antibody produced in response to the vaccine in the Taiji group when compared to controls, the intervention failed to stimulate antibody production above a critical level (e.g. ≥ 40 HI) needed for protection against influenza infection [14]. Although there were some differences across the vaccine strains, there was a tendency for the intervention to increase the percentage of people exhibiting a protective titer >40 HI, although this was not statistically significant.

There are a few limitations to this study that are noteworthy. First, this was intended as a proof of concept study and was not a true randomized controlled trial. We were unsuccessful in recruiting enough control subjects (n = 14) from the larger parent trial to effectively compare the efficacy of the intervention (n = 27) on influenza vaccine responses. As such, we recruited additional subjects (n = 9) to the wait-list control group in a nonrandomized fashion. We made every attempt to make sure that these subjects were similar to the parent trial by using the same inclusion/exclusion criteria. Our results indicated that on most variables (e.g. gender, BMI, number of medications, diagnosed diseases, exercise participation, vitamin and alcohol use) the two groups were comparable. The only borderline significant (p = 0.05) difference was in age. The TQ group was on average 5.5 years older than the control group. However, older age results in reduced influenza vaccine responsiveness [13], suggesting a possible underestimation of the TQ effects reported in the current study. A second limitation of the present study was our lack of an attention control group. This limited our ability to determine whether the increase in antibody titer seen in the TQ group was due to the behavioral Taiji intervention or socialization into the study. Third, while we made every attempt to ascertain each participant's previous year's (2002–2003; which was identical to the 2003–2004 vaccine used in the current study) influenza vaccine exposure, a few of our subjects could not recall whether they had or had not received that vaccine. In the 92% who could recall, there were no significant differences in the percentage receiving the vaccine in the TQ (50%) when compared to the controls (60%). We also found no differences in baseline titers to any of the strains (table 1) and, importantly, our statistical model adjusted baselines between the groups to examine relative change over time. Thus, we are confident that group differences in the response to the influenza vaccine used in this study were due to factors other than prior exposure. Lastly, while anti-influenza antibodies generated in response to vaccine are important in influenza prevention, cell-mediated immune responses also play a role [13]. Indeed, a recent study suggests that T cell-mediated responses mounted in response to the influenza vaccine may be more predictive of vaccine protection in the elderly when compared to antibody responses [15]. We did not assess the cell-mediated immune response to the vaccine in the present study. Despite these limitations, studies such as this one provide evidence for mind-body interactions and demonstrate the utility of such behavioral interventions as complementary therapy for those whose immune systems operate suboptimally. Clearly, there needs to be a large, randomized controlled trial on TQ intervention and vaccine efficacy in this at-risk population.

There have been some studies that have examined the effects of Taiji and Qigong on immune function in various populations. Unfortunately, few of these studies have included clinically relevant measures of immunocompetence and several are inadequately controlled. For example, Manzaneque et al. [16] found that 1 month of Qigong training lowered total leukocyte, eosinophil, monocyte and complement C3 levels. Jones [17] found that 14 weeks of Guolin Qigong increased the IFN-γ:IL-10 ratio in leukocytes cultured with phytohemagglutinin in vitro. The lack of a control group in this study made it difficult to assess the contribution of the intervention. Moreover, simple measures of leukocyte counts or ex vivo cytokine production in response to polyclonal stimulation have little clinical relevance. In one carefully controlled clinically relevant trial, Irwin et al. [10] found that 15 weeks of a Westernized version of Taiji significantly increase varicella zoster virus-specific immunity in men and women aged over 60. Also, it has been found that Qigong-trained subjects mounted better responses to delayed-type hypersensitivity recall antigens when compared to controls [18]. The latter is clinically relevant because low delayed-type hypersensitivity responses have been found to be related to higher mortality due to sepsis [19]. Although not Taiji, mindfulness meditation techniques have resulted in improved antibody titers to influenza vaccine in a group of younger subjects [20]. Recent evidence also suggests that physical exercise can improve the antibody response to influenza vaccination in previously sedentary elderly [21]. This effect was mediated, in part, by improvements in psychosocial factors [22, 23], which unfortunately we did not assess in the present study.

While the underlying mechanisms behind behavioral intervention's beneficial effects on immune responsiveness in some studies remains unclear, it is well known that there exist established links between behavior and neuroendocrine factors that can impact immune cells. For example, immune cells express adrenergic and cholinergic receptors and catecholamines and acetylcholine have profound effects on their functions [24, 25]. Interestingly, Taijiquan (T'ai Chi Chuan) has been found to enhance vagal modulation and shift the sympathovagal balance towards a reduction in sympathetic tone [26]. Whether changes in autonomic balance in response to behavioral interventions like Taiji are responsible for altered immune responsiveness to challenge is unknown, but testable. This is the first study adopting a traditional curriculum

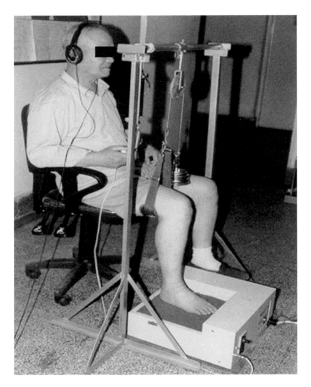

Fig. 1. Testing apparatus and a subject positioning for evaluation of passive motion sense of ankle joint.

Measurement

Each subject individually participated in two separate sessions of data collection. The first one was measurement of ankle joint kinesthesia. After a brief rest period, knee joint kinesthesia was tested.

Ankle Joint Kinesthesia Test

Data were collected using the instrumentation and procedures described by Lentell et al. [13], but small changes were instituted. As illustrated in figure 1, the custom-made device is a box with a movable platform that rotates about a single axis in two directions. With the foot resting on this platform, plantar-dorsiflexion of ankle movements can occur. This platform is moved by an electric motor that rotates the foot on an axis at a rate of 0.4°/s. Movement can be stopped at any time with the use of a hand-held switch. The angular motion achieved by the platform is calculated by the dents that the motor rotates.

The device is also equipped with a hanging scale and a fixed pulley supported by a trestle, which is outside of the device. A thigh cuff attached to the lower end of the scale is wrapped around the lower thigh of the subjects. Through adjusting the length of the cuff, the extremity is lifted by the scale and its weight is recorded when the subjects fully relax their thigh. After this, the thigh cuff is attached to one end of the rope around the pulley and the other end is hung with weights. The extremity can then be adjusted to where the foot is in contact with the platform. Through adding or reducing the weights, the investigator can standardize the weight of the lower extremity resting on the platform during testing.

For data collection, each subject was seated on an adjustable chair and his or her dominant foot was so placed on the platform that the axis of the apparatus coincided with the plantar-dorsiflexion axis of the ankle joint. The hip, knee, and ankle were positioned at 90° respectively. In order to standardize the sensory cues from the contact between the instrument and the plantar surface of the foot, 50% of each subject's lower extremity weight was rested on the platform by the use of the thigh cuff suspension system. During testing, the subjects' eyes were closed and they wore headphones with music playing to eliminate visual and auditory stimuli from the testing procedure apparatus.

Each test movement began with the foot placed on the horizontal platform, namely the starting position was 0°. The subjects were instructed to concentrate on their foot and to press the hand switch when they could sense motion and identify the direction of the movement. After performing two practice trials, the motor was then engaged to rotate the foot into dorsiflexion or plantarflexion at a random time interval between 2 and 10 s after subject instruction. The researcher recorded the rotation angles of the platform and the direction of movements as passive motion sense. At least six randomized trials were conducted: three for plantarflexion, three for dorsiflexion. The mean values of three trials in one direction were calculated.

Knee Joint Kinesthesia Test

The method of assessing knee kinesthesia was similar to those described in previous studies [2, 14]. As shown in figure 2, the apparatus consists of electric motor, governor, counter system, transmission and linkage system. A moveable frame can rotate around a single axis in two directions at a velocity of 0.4°/s. Angular displacement of the frame is calculated by the dents that the motor rotates.

Each subject performed two practice tests to become familiar with the test process before completing the trials. At least six randomized trials (three trials for extension, three trials for flexion) were tested in his or her dominant leg according to the following protocol. The subjects wore shorts to negate any extraneous skin sensation from clothing through the knee area. They sat in an adjustable chair with the legs hanging freely over the edge of the seat 5 cm proximal to the popliteal fossa. A custom-made inflatable cuff was fitted above the knee joint and inflated to 20 mm Hg to neutralize cutaneous sensation. The axis of rotation of the knee joint was aligned with the axis of rotation of the frame. Then the researcher placed the lower part of the shank of the subject on the frame. An ankle inflatable cuff was applied and inflated to 20 mm Hg to reduce multisensory afferent discharge at the shank-machine interface. To further reduce unwanted sensory input, the subjects kept their eyes closed and wore headphones with music playing to eliminate the sight and sound of the apparatus.

The starting position of each trial was 45° of knee flexion as measured by an electrogoniometer (Penny and Giles, Christchurch, UK). Subjects were told that their legs could move in a flexed or extended direction beginning at a random delay of 2–10 s after the examiner signaled the start of the test. Once the subject detected motion of the leg, he or she pressed a handheld stop button and confirmed the direction of the motion. The rotation angles of the

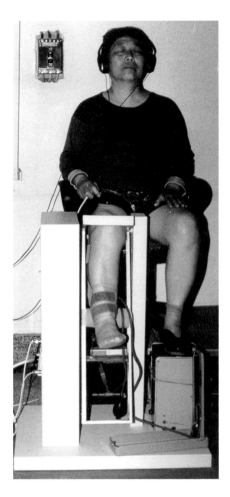

Fig. 2. Customized apparatus used to test passive motion sense of knee joint.

frame were defined as the threshold for detection of the knee joint. Mean values of three trials in one direction were used for analysis.

Data Analysis

All variables were presented as means and standard deviations. Passive motion sense of ankle and knee joint in different directions were respectively compared using paired t test in each group. Because there were no significant differences between the directions of ankle movement, plantarflexion and dorsiflexion data were averaged to present the ankle kinesthesia. One-way analysis of variance was used to estimate significant differences among groups. The post-hoc Scheffe tests were performed when necessary to isolate the differences and $p \leq 0.05$ was considered statistically significant.

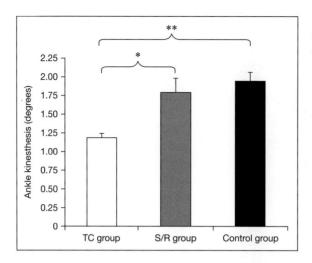

Fig. 3. Comparison of ankle kinesthesis in the TC, S/R and control groups. Error bar indicates standard error of mean (SEM). **p < 0.01, *p < 0.05 compared with the TC group.

Results

Ankle Joint Kinesthesia

Ankle joint kinesthesia significantly differed among the three groups (p $= 0.001$). Movements of 1.21 $\pm$ 0.33° were perceived in the TC group, 1.78 $\pm$ 0.82° in the S/R group, and 1.95 $\pm$ 0.66° in the sedentary control group. The post-hoc test showed that TC practitioners could detect a significantly smaller amount of motion than the sedentary counterparts (p $= 0.001$) and swimming/running exercisers (p $= 0.022$), while no significant difference was found between the S/R group and sedentary control group (p $= 0.701$; fig. 3).

Knee Joint Kinesthesia

The threshold for detection of passive motion was significantly different in the knee extension and flexion of each group; the knees were more sensitive to a flexion arc than they were to an extension arc. One-way ANOVA analysis indicated that significant differences in passive motion sense were evident in

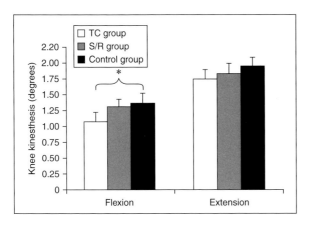

Fig. 4. Comparison of knee kinesthesis in the TC S/R control groups. Error bar indicates standard error of mean (SEM). *p < 0.05 compared with the TC group.

knee flexion across the three groups (p = 0.025). Further analysis showed that the TC group had a significantly smaller mean threshold for detection of passive motion than did the subjects in the control group (p = 0.026). There were no significant differences between the S/R group and the control group (p = 0.312), the TC group and S/R group (p = 0.533). For knee extension, no significant difference was found among the three groups (p = 0.597; fig. 4).

Discussion

Although many studies have indicated that the adaptation of regular physical activity can certainly attenuate the age-related decline in many physiologic systems, few of them have been concerned about the effects of exercise on proprioception of old people, especially for the effects of different kinds of exercise. Our study provided evidence that long-term TC practitioners not only showed better ankle and knee joint kinesthesia than sedentary controls but also their ankle joint kinesthesia was better than the long-term swimming/running exercisers. Furthermore, the latter did not perform better in ankle and knee joint kinesthesis test than their sedentary counterparts.

The movements of TC are gracefully fluent and consummately precise because specificity of joint angles and body position is of critical importance in accurately and correctly performing each form [15]. Acute awareness of body position and movement is demanded by the nature of the activity. Thus TC practice might have more benefits for proprioception. The findings of the present study identified this characteristic.

Swimming and running are two of the most common exercises practiced by elderly people, which are excellent forms of aerobic exercise, and provide good training stimuli for the cardiopulmonary function and muscle strength. Compared with TC exercise, swimming or running is a kind of cyclic repetitive action. The awareness of joint position and movement is not specially emphasized during these exercise forms. Additionally, most elderly people exercise only for enhancing health and recreation; they usually do not pay much attention to joint position and angles during exercise, unless the awareness of the joint position and angles is specially required in some exercises, such as TC. This might be one of the reasons that swimming/running exercisers did not show the better scores in the measurements of knee and ankle kinesthesia in this study.

Of particular interest in this study, the impact of TC practice on proprioception was different in knee and ankle joints. Its effect on ankle joint kinesthesia was more prominent than that on knee joint kinesthesia. The passive motion sense of the ankle joint in the TC group was not only significantly better than that in sedentary control group but also than that in swimming/running group. However, for the knee joint TC exercise only produced a better effect than the sedentary control group. These results might be attributed to the characteristics of TC movements. The old TC proverb states, 'When performing TC, the feet act as roots'. Although almost all TC forms are performed in semi-squat position, which enhances the loading of muscles and motion ranges of knee joints, the continuous transformation of different postures and steps causes more changes of ankle joint movements, such as turning tocs outward or inward, raising toes or putting down and so on. Moreover, while making stride foot placement is slow and deliberate. These movements might be of benefit for retaining proprioceptor's sensitivity located in the joint capsules, ligaments, tendons and muscles.

The ankle proprioception is very important for the elderly to maintain proper postural control. Many studies have indicated that a movement pattern for postural correction in elderly adults is different from that of young adults. The elderly rely more on hip movements while the young people rely on ankle movements to control postural stability [16]. Decline of somatosensory information from feet is one of the major factors pertaining to this pattern change with age [17]. Therefore, the considerable impact of TC practice on ankle proprioception was very beneficial for old people to retain balance control.

Decline in proprioception with age may be an important contributing factor to falls in the elderly, and this may be influenced by regular physical activity.

The current study demonstrated that compared with other common activities, long-term TC exercise produced more beneficial effects on retaining the old people's proprioception in ankle and knee joints, which may be helpful to maintain balance control in the elderly.

Conclusion

For the ankle joint, TC practitioners could detect a significantly smaller amount of motion than S/R exercisers and sedentary counterparts. For the knee joint, the TC group showed a significantly smaller mean threshold for detection of passive motion in knee flexion compared with the control group.

Acknowledgements

The work described in this paper was fully supported by a grant from the Research Grants Council of the Hong Kong Special Administrative Region (project CUHK4360/00H).

References

1   Lephart SM, Pincivero DM, Giraldo JL, et al: The role of proprioception in the management and rehabilitation of athletic injuries. Am J Sports Med 1997;25:130–137.
2   Pai YC, Rymer WZ, Chang RW, et al: Effect of age and osteoarthritis on knee proprioception. Arthritis Rheum 1997;40:2260–2265.
3   Petrella RJ, Lattanzio PJ, Nelson MG: Effect of age and activity on knee joint proprioception. Am J Phys Med Rehabil 1997;76:235–241.
4   Skinner HB, Barrack RL, Cook SD: Age-related decline in proprioception. Clin Orthop Rel Res 1984;184:208–211.
5   Robbins S, Waked E, McClaran J: Proprioception and stability: foot position awareness as a function of age and footwear. Age Ageing 1995;24:67–72.
6   Mion LC, Gregor S, Buettner M, et al: Falls in the rehabilitation setting: incidence and characteristics. Rehabil Nurs 1989;14:17–22.
7   Lord SR, Ward JA, William P, et al: Physiological factors associated with falls in older community-dwelling women. J Am Geriatr 1994;42:17–21.
8   Lord SR, Rogers MS, Howland A, et al: Lateral stability, sensorimotor function and falls in older prople. J Am Geriatr 1999;47:1077–1081.
9   Gauchard GC, Jeandel C, Tessier A, et al: Beneficial effect of proprioceptive physical activities on balance control in elderly human subjects. Neurosci Lett 1999;273:81–84.
10 Hong Y, Li JX, Robinson PD: Balance control, flexibility, and cardiorespiratory fitness among older Tai Chi practitioners. Br J Sports Med 2000;34:29–34.
11 Tse SK, Bailey DM: T'ai chi and postural control in the well elderly. Am J Occup Thera 1992;46:295–300.
12 Wolf SL, Barnhart HX, Kutner NG, et al: Reducing frailty and falls in older persons: An investigation of Tai Chi and computerized balance training. J Am Geriatr Soc 1996;44:489–497.
13 Lentell G, Baas B, Lopez D, et al: The contributions of proprioceptive deficits, muscle function, and anatomic laxity to functional instability of the ankle. JOSPT 1995;21:206–215.

14   Beynnon BD, Renstrom PA, Konradsen L, et al: Validation of techniques to measure knee propri-
      oception; in Lephart SM, Fu FH (eds): Proprioception and Neuromuscular Control in Joint Stabil-
      ity. United States: Human Kinetics, 2000, pp 127–138.
15   Jacobson BH, Chen HC, Cashel C, et al: The effect of Tai Chi Chuan training on balance, kines-
      thetic sense, and strength. Percept Mot Skills 1997;84:27–33.
16   Okada S, Hirakawa K, Takada Y, et al: Age-related differences in postural control in humans in
      response to a sudden deceleration generated by postural disturbance. Eur J Appl Physiol 2001;
      85:10–18.
17   Manchester D, Woollacott M, Zederbauer-Hylton N, et al: Visual, vestibular and somatosensory
      contributions to balance control in the older adult. J Gerontol 1989;44:M118–M127.

Prof. Jing Xian Li, PhD
School of Human Kinetics, University of Ottawa
125 University Street
Ottawa, Ontario, K1N-6N5 (Canada)
Tel. +1 613 562 5800 Ext. 2457, Fax +1 613 562 5149, E-Mail jli@uottawa.ca

Hong Y (ed): Tai Chi Chuan. State of the Art in International Research.
Med Sport Sci. Basel, Karger, 2008, vol 52, pp 87–103

....

Neural Mechanisms Underlying Balance Control in Tai Chi

Strawberry Gatts

Clinical Biomechanics and Rehabilitation Lab., Department of Kinesiology, College
of Applied Health Sciences, University of Illinois at Chicago, Chicago, Ill., USA

Abstract

Background and Aims: The efficacy of Tai Chi (TC) to improve neuromuscular
response characteristics underlying dynamic balance recovery in balance-impaired seniors at
high risk for falling was examined during perturbed walking. **Methods:** Twenty-two subjects
were randomized into TC or control groups. Nineteen subjects (68–92 years, BERG 44 or less)
completed the study. TC training incorporated repetitive exercises using TC's essential
motor/biomechanical strategies, techniques, and postural components. Control training used
axial exercises, balance awareness/education and stress reduction. Groups trained 1.5 h/day,
5 days/week for 3 weeks. After post-testing, controls received TC training. Subjects walked
across a force plate triggered to move forward 15 cm at 40 cm/s at heelstrike. Tibialis anterior
and medial gastrocnemius responses during balance recovery were recorded from electromyograms. Four clinical measures of balance were also examined. **Results:** TC subjects, but not
controls, significantly reduced tibialis anterior response time from 148.92 ± 45.11 ms to
98.67 ± 17.22 ms ($p \leq 0.004$) and decreased cocontraction of antagonist muscles ($p \leq 0.003$)
of the perturbed leg. All clinical balance measures significantly improved after TC.
Conclusions: TC training transferred to improved neuromuscular responses controlling the
ankle joint during perturbed gait in balance-impaired seniors who had surgical interventions to
their back, hips, knees and arthritis. The fast, accurate neuromuscular activation crucial for efficacious response to slips also transferred to four clinical measures of functional balance.
Significant enhancement was achieved with 3 weeks of training.

Copyright © 2008 S. Karger AG, Basel

A variety of studies concerning Tai Chi's (TC) effects on balance control in
older adults have been performed, and many showed that TC reduced fall risk and
improved balance in older adults [1–5]. Though these studies indicated TC
improved senior's balance, the mechanisms underlying this improvement were not
clear, and it is unknown which recovery mechanisms were most affected.

Additionally, no TC studies have, to date, examined reactive balance control during gait in seniors at high-risk for falling [6]. Consequently, it would be most informative to examine specific neuromuscular mechanisms before and after TC training and compare the results to a similar but different training given to a control group. Additionally, in order to adequately identify if the intervention training transfers to dynamic balance recovery, there is a need to use a testing paradigm that mimics real world balance challenges. Lastly, it would be informative to train older subjects that represent the general population that balance programs would need to address, i.e. seniors with multiple sources of balance deficits.

The most common situation encountered by the elderly which leads to falling is tripping or slipping while walking forward, followed by falling during transfer and falling on stairs or steps [7]. Balance recovery during walking is a dynamic process requiring the ability to make rapid, coordinated, and accurate modifications to body posture to prevent falling. Given that an inability to recover from a slip or trip during walking accounts for the majority of falls in seniors, it would be most informative to examine the effects of balance interventions during a slip/trip while walking. Thus, the dynamics of the recovery process required by real world activities suggests that assessments, interventions and test measures using sudden perturbations during gait are necessary to truly evaluate balance control. Furthermore, therapeutic interventions would likely benefit by incorporating balance skill training that practices controlling a variety of spatial and temporal changes during a dynamic movement such as gait.

Previously, Tang and Woollacott [8] investigated neuromuscular mechanisms underlying age-related declines in balance reactions by 'slipping' young or healthy older subjects using a forward platform movement. The platform slid 10 cm forward at 40 cm/s at heelstrike. Postural muscle responses were recorded from electromyograms (EMGs). They hypothesized older adults would use a less effective reactive balance strategy than young adults. Results indicated that, compared to young adults, older adults' postural muscle responses were characterized by: (1) increased coactivation of agonist and antagonist muscles; (2) longer contraction onset time, and (3) longer muscle burst durations.

Our present study [9] used a similar test paradigm to determine the effects of TC training on neuromuscular response characteristics underlying balance control in balance-impaired seniors at high risk for falling. We did, however, lengthen the distance of the slip to 15 cm. We compared training effects after TC to a control group given a similar intensity training using axial exercises, stretching, stress reduction, and awareness/balance education. We hypothesized that neural mechanisms contributing to improvements after TC training would include: (1) decreased time to tibialis anterior (TA) muscle contraction onset in response to the perturbation, (2) improved organization of muscle responses and (3) reduced cocontraction of antagonist muscles during postural adjustments.

We also hypothesized TC training would transfer to an improved performance on four commonly used clinical tests of functional balance control: Functional Reach (FR), Timed Up and GO (TUG), One leg stance time, and Tandem stance time.

Previous TC studies differed from the present study in five ways. To date, TC interventions did not include balance-impaired older adults with multiple surgical interventions to their back, hips and/or knees. Because it is likely that interventions for balance-impaired older populations would include such individuals, we did not exclude this population. Second, previous TC studies relied heavily on standing balance measures [1–6] whereas our study examined neuromuscular responses during a large/fast slip during locomotion. Third, studies did not compare differences in balance responses in the same subjects after two different interventions. Our control group was given the TC intervention after completing control training. This crossover design allowed us to explore neuromuscular responses before and after two interventions in the same subjects. Fourth, previous TC research [1–6] used TC postural sequences. Our intervention focused on the use of TC principles (motor and biomechanical techniques and postural elements) to control dynamic balance rather than performing a sequence of postures. Fifth, past studies did not examine a short (3 weeks) intensified training that better suits clinical and therapeutic environments.

Our study was conducted to determine how fall-recovery mechanisms were affected by TC balance training in aging populations at high risk for falls [9, 10]. Our long-term goals include further development of training and assessment programs for mobility-impaired populations, applying TC training principles to the design of robotic and mechanical training aids and to training protocols that enhance reflexive motor skills, injury prevention, and team performance for sports and industry.

Methods

Clinical Measures

Control and TC groups received identical clinical testing before and after training. Scores evaluated before each type of training served as the pretest for post-training comparison. FR [11], TUG [12], single right/left leg stance, tandem stance right/left leg behind were chosen because they are common clinical tests used to assess balance skills in older adults [13], and they could be quantified.

Tests were demonstrated by the examiner until participants clearly understood the task. Data from the first trial the participant was able to perform were recorded because our study focused on change in the initial recovery response. Maximum time recorded for single and tandem stance tests was 30 s [2]. Subjects with maximum scores of 30 s were scored with the value of 30 s. The difference score of subjects with scores of 30 s at pre- and post-training was 0. Single stance time was recorded from the right and left leg separately. Tandem stance was tested once with the right leg in front and once with the left leg in front. In order to have comparable responses on clinical and laboratory tests, we used the initial score for TUG and FR, although this departs from normal testing procedures. Participants were tested barefoot or in stocking feet.

Functional Reach

FR examines limits of stability in the forward direction [14] and is related to range of motion in the axial spinal column. It is sensitive to change after exercise [15]. Subjects were directed to stand with feet shoulder-width apart and raise their right arm to $90°$ in front. The distance they were able to lean forward without moving their feet was recorded in inches.

Timed Up and Go

TUG is related to functional capacity measured by the Barthel Index [16]. Seated subjects stood up from a chair, walked 3 m at normal speed, turned around, returned to the chair and sat down. Performance was timed in seconds with a stopwatch.

Single Stance Time

This is a demanding task for stability because the body's center of mass must balance on a narrow base of support. Due its difficulty, it has become the most frequently used measure of balance in studies of older adults [17]. Subjects stood with eyes open on one leg and raised the other leg above the ground. The number of seconds the subject maintained balance without touching the ground with the elevated foot or grabbing a support was recorded. Maximum time recorded was 30 s [2, 17].

Tandem Stance Time

Subjects stood unsupported with one foot placed so that the heel of the forward foot was in front of the toe of the back foot and both feet formed a straight line [2]. This is a bipedal variation of single stance. Maximum time recorded was 30 s.

Subjects

Subjects were invited to the University of Oregon Motor Control lab after they had passed a phone interview. Participation criteria were 65 years or older, diagnosed as balance-impaired by their physician or physical therapist, Berg balance score of 45 or less [18], no diagnosed neurological disorders, able to stand without support and cognitively able to follow instructions. Those with arthritis, back, knee, or hip surgery were not excluded because these subjects represented the real world population that balance interventions need to address. Subjects lived independently in the community and drove or rode a bus to training or test sites. Each participant signed an informed consent approved by the Committee for the Protection of Human Subjects/Institutional Review Board of the University of Oregon and conformed to the standards set by the Declaration of Helsinki.

Participants (n = 22) were randomly divided into TC or control groups. Nineteen subjects (68–92 years, mean 77.55) completed the study. Three female subjects were dropped from the control group (2 wanted only TC training and 1 declined testing on the platform).

Table 1. Demographics of the groups

Subject No.	Gender	Age	Height, cm	Mass, kg	Berg	TUG, s	FR, inches
Group 1							
1	F	75.0	165.0	69.5	42.0	13.79	8.0
2	F	68.0	164.0	75.2	30.0	10.04	9.5
3	F	75.0	162.0	94.0	24.0	13.03	10.0
4	F	92.0	169.0	61.5	41.0	15.66	13.0
5	F	81.0	156.0	66.0	41.0	12.55	10.0
6	F	82.0	167.0	71.0	38.0	14.69	6.0
7	F	76.0	164.0	70.5	41.0	11.30	9.0
8	M	71.0	165.0	66.0	42.0	11.70	11.0
9	F	86.0	149.5	61.0	33.0	18.31	6.0
10	F	73.0	156.0	71.5	40.0	10.09	9.0
11	F	75.0	162.0	63.5	42.0	12.58	8.0
Mean		77.6	161.8	70.0	37.6	13.07	9.05
SD		7.0	5.7	9.1	6.02	2.47	2.05
Groups 2a and 2b							
12	F	68.0	170.00	75.5	40.0	12.27	9.00
13	F	80.0	160.00	80.0	36.0	12.80	6.00
14	F	82.0	163.00	58.0	41.0	10.06	6.25
15	F	81.0	159.00	69.5	44.0	12.62	10.50
16	F	85.0	164.00	69.0	28.0	18.47	4.50
17	M	75.0	179.00	98.0	44.0	12.05	6.50
18	F	73.0	149.00	67.0	39.0	13.00	12.00
19	F	76.0	164.00	88.5	28.0	15.85	12.00
Mean		77.5	163.50	75.7	37.5	13.39	8.34
SD		5.5	8.70	12.8	6.41	2.59	2.92

Group 1 and groups 2a and 2b were similar in age ($p = 0.96$), height ($p = 0.63$), mass ($p = 0.30$), and impairment (arthritis: $p = 0.15$; surgery to spine: $p = 0.41$, knee: $p = 0.75$, or hip: $p = 0.17$), Berg ($p = 0.96$), TUG ($p = 0.79$), FR ($p = 0.57$). Reprinted with permission from Gatts and Woollacott [9].

One control (14) did not complete crossover training because of a family emergency. Groups (table 1) were similar in age ($p = 0.96$), height ($p = 0.63$), mass ($p = 0.30$), and impairment (arthritis, $p = 0.15$; spinal surgery, $p = 0.41$; knee surgery, $p = 0.75$; hip replacement, $p = 0.17$; Berg, $p = 0.96$, TUG, $p = 0.79$; FR, $p = 0.57$).

Interventions

Training was 1.5 h/day, 5 days/week for 3 weeks in local community centers. Groups received similar times for exercise and discussion. Pre-testing for each group took place during the week before training and post-testing the week after. Average time between testing was 4 weeks.

Tai Chi

We used classical TC training techniques, which differ from previous reports of TC interventions. Traditional methods first perform well-coordinated sequencing of change (flow) within a standing posture before progressing to walking postures or linking postures into sequences. This stage involves learning to control and integrate several TC principles: accurate center of mass and segmental positioning, muscle force control, flowing oscillation (as opposed to jerking), and dynamic balance control during changes in the configuration of the base of support. Each principle was first practiced individually. Next, principles were combined one by one so that a growing number of principles melded within a single exercise/posture. During the next stage a complete TC posture was practiced bilaterally during stance. Once postures were performed accurately during stance, TC gait was added. Each posture and gesture was carefully practiced individually so the students could seek to correct their mistakes and gain the benefit of the practice [19]. Dr. Gatts, who trained in TC full time for 9 years with Chinese masters and has taught TC since 1984, based the TC intervention on her work with over 6,000 adults, most of whom had balance/mobility deficits.

The following TC postures were used: Commencement, White Stork Cools its Wing, Brush Knee, Play the Guitar/Play the Harp, Repulse the Monkey, Heel Kick, Toe Kick, Golden Cockerel, Fair Lady Works the Shuttles, Part the Wild Horses' Mane, Cloud Hands, Cross Hands. *Tai Chi Chuan: The 27 Forms* [20], researched and ghostwritten by Dr. Gatts, lists the health benefits of each posture.

Controls

Control training included components theoretically similar to TC training: awareness and balance education, stress reduction, deep breathing, and axial exercise. Awareness education covered age-related changes in sensory, neuromuscular, biomechanical and cognitive systems and how such changes can lead to decreased balance control and reduced ability to simultaneously attend to multiple factors. Techniques and strategies to increase sensory awareness of fall onset, factors contributing to falls or near falls and useful recovery strategies were also covered [17, 21, 22]. Balance education included environmental and home safety information [21, 23, 24]. Exercise, deep breathing, stress reduction, and tension control components used the Axial Exercise Program [25] and the Guide to Fitness After Fifty [26]. Axial exercises were chosen because they were designed to improve postural alignment, increase range of motion, coordinate relaxed movement as opposed to effort, relax tight muscles using deep breathing, use muscle groups with appropriate mechanical advantage, and enhance participation of appropriate synergistic muscles used in activities of daily living. Controls received TC training after post-control training testing.

Lab Procedures

Subjects participated in identical lab sessions before and after training and were tested barefoot or in stocking feet. Since previous research indicated adaptations to platform perturbations can occur by the third trial [27], we analyzed responses from the first trial because this was analogous to a real life slip where we do not have a chance to 'do it again'. Berger et al. [28] have shown EMG responses were unaltered by pre-warning or random onset of the perturbation. Therefore, we told our high-risk population that the forceplate would move forward 15 cm. Subjects walked at self-selected speed. Data were collected for 6 s. An overhead suspension cable was attached to a body harness worn by the subject.

The slip was induced as subjects walked across a custom-built force platform constructed of two metal platforms (1.84 m long × 0.51 m wide × 0.35 m high) incorporated into the center of a 5 m long × 1.10 m wide × 0.35 m high wooden walkway. A moveable force plate (0.61 m long × 0.17 m wide) was placed in the center of each platform. The left plate remained stationary while the right plate moved 15 cm forward at 40 cm/sec. This velocity was chosen because it matched reported horizontal heel velocities on slippery surfaces during realistic slips [29]. Plate movement was triggered by a 40-newton Fz force signal from the right heel strike connected to a PC via a D–A converter. Analog data (EMG and force platform data) were collected with a data acquisition system (AMLAB, Australia). All data were analyzed from the onset of actual plate movement.

EMG surface electrodes MA-300 from Motion Lab Systems, Inc. (Baton Rouge, La., USA) recorded neuromuscular responses. Electrodes were placed on the right TA, right medial gastrocnemius (GA) and on the ulna head of the wrist (ground). Electrode output went to a preamp/power supply attached to a vest worn by the subject. Common-mode rejection ratio was >100 dB at 40 Hz. EMG signal output was ±5 V full scale. Raw analog EMG signals were on-line preamplified (gain 4,000) and analog filtered (20–2,000 Hz), then converted into digital signals sampled at 1,200 HZ for 6 s. A built-in low-pass analog filter was set at 600 Hz.

Custom-written programs in MATLAB (The MathWorks, Natick, Mass., USA) were used for further data processing. EMG signals were full-wave rectified and low-pass filtered using a fourth order dual-pass Butterworth filter prior to analysis. Cutoff frequency was 50 Hz. Plate onset time was determined as the time the plate registered 3 standard deviations (SD) above its stationary position. Baseline muscle activity was computed for each muscle by averaging its summed activity for 500 ms before plate onset. EMG activity was computed and graphed for 50 ms before plate onset to 1,800 ms after plate onset. EMG activity in each muscle was computed for pre- to post-differences for: cocontraction of the agonist/antagonist, muscle burst duration, muscle onset latency, reversed activation (GA onset preceded TA onset), and percent muscle burst duration (to account for differences in walking speed).

Cocontraction was the time the TA and GA were simultaneously active longer than 10 ms during muscle burst duration. Burst duration was defined as time between muscle onset and offset, with offset defined as the time at which muscle activity fell below 2 SD for longer than 30 ms. Muscle onset latency was the time between plate onset and the time when muscle activity increased 2 SD above baseline. Reversed activation was defined as a trial during which GA onset preceded TA onset. Percent duration was defined as the percent of time a muscle was active while the right foot remained on the plate.

Analysis

PROC MIXED from SAS software was used to run a one-way analysis of covariance (ANCOVA) to evaluate pre-post differences in clinical measures. PROC MEANS from SAS software was used to run a t test examining each lab measure one at a time. Results were compared with nonparametric tests from PROC UNIVARIATE. Muscle response organization

Table 2. Main effects of training on clinical measures

Measure	Group 1			Group 2a			Group 2b		
	mean	SE	p	mean	SE	p	mean	SE	p
Timed Up and Go, s	3.53	0.49	0.0001	0.08	0.57	0.8949	3.02	0.62	0.0001
FR, inches	3.31	0.63	0.0001	2.90	0.77	0.0011	4.22	0.93	0.0002
Stand on right leg, s	13.06	3.25	0.0007	0.19	3.65	0.9583	9.65	4.00	0.0260
Stand on left leg, s	12.58	2.41	0.0001	0.30	2.63	0.9101	4.11	2.83	0.1644
Tandem stance right leg behind, s	12.79	3.00	0.0004	0.004	3.44	0.9991	8.20	3.85	0.0452
Tandem stance left leg behind, s	12.81	3.00	0.0003	2.27	3.42	0.5133	9.84	3.85	0.0182

Least square means from ANCOVA model with main effects for group. Mean and standard error (SE) are based on the pre-post difference scores. $p \leq 0.05$ for main effect. Group 1 = TC only; Group 2 = crossover group (controls 2a, TC 2b). Reprinted with permission from Gatts and Woollacott [9].

and occurrence of cocontraction were measured with two outcomes: correct (agonist contracts before antagonist muscle, 10 ms or less overlap of the TA and GA muscle bursts)/incorrect (antagonist contracts before agonist, 10 ms or more overlap of the TA and GA muscle bursts). Accounting for the correlated structure of responses across test periods, logistic regression coefficients were computed to estimate odds of a correct response in each group and then compared the odds ratio of the treatment group with the control group. PROC GENMOD of SAS was used, as it allowed choosing an appropriate covariance structure. Exact Pearson χ^2 test, designed for small cell counts, examined the effect of time. An exact logistic regression test examined training effects. Additional statistical details can be found in Gatts and Woollacott [9].

Results

Table 2 shows main effects of training for each clinical measure. TC groups improved significantly on most tests while controls significantly improved only on FR. Interestingly, after TC, control subjects were able to significantly improve their FR distance by an additional 4.22 inches.

Table 3 shows main training effects for each neuromuscular measure. TC subjects (group 1 and 2b) significantly reduced TA onset times, but controls (group 2a) did not (fig. 1a). TA muscle burst duration did not change significantly in any group after training. GA onset changed significantly after training only in TC group 2b and was chiefly due to 2 subjects taking 282 and

Table 3. Main effects of training on TA and GA measures

Measure	Group 1			Group 2a			Group 2b		
	Mean	SD	p	Mean	SD	p	Mean	SD	p
TA onset 1, ms	148.92	45.11		136.42	73.21		104.98	25.58	
TA onset 2, ms	98.67	17.22	≤0.004*	104.15	23.8	≤0.138	87.62	10.19	≤0.028*
TA duration 1, ms	158.95	105.60		223.27	92.61		158.33	82.15	
TA duration 2, ms	161.50	63.70	≤0.473	165.52	78.73	≤0.099	144.76	65.45	≤0.400
TA duration 1, %[1]	15	12		20	9		18	8	
TA duration 2, %[1]	17	7	≤0.298	19	8	≤0.426	17	9	≤0.451
GA onset 1, ms	349.49	168.90		328.75	242.99		238.81	87.52	
GA onset 2, ms	316.93	66.43	≤0.310	242.81	81.31	≤0.173	380.95	119.74	≤0.025*
GA duration 1, ms	246.97	120.50		325.88	278.74		242.86	253.2	
GA duration 2, ms	88.93	68.55	≤0.002*	223.23	240.9	≤0.060	166.9	126.19	≤0.250
GA duration 1, %[1]	22	14		27	22		27	25	
GA duration 2, %[1]	10	8	≤0.012*	25	24	≤0.340	21	17	≤0.300
Subjects reversed 1, %[2]	33			50			14.30		
Subjects reversed 2, %[2]	0		≤0.105	12.5		≤0.128	0		≤0.500
Cocontraction 1, ms	60.33	80.15		119.90	123.58		60.81	113.52	
Cocontraction 2, ms	0.50	1.58		58.63	105.28		0.00	0.00	
Subject with cocontraction 1, %[2]	60			63			43		
Subjects with cocontraction 2, %[2]	0		≤0.016*	50		≤0.192	0		≤0.096

*p ≤ 0.05 (paired-sample t tests, one-tailed). 1 designates pre-test and 2 designates post-test. Reprinted with permission from Gatts and Woollacott [9].

[1] Normalized muscle activity as a percent of time the muscle is active while the foot remains on the plate accounts for possible differences in walking velocity.

[2] An odds ratio was used to compare odds of the event occurring at time 1 and time 2.

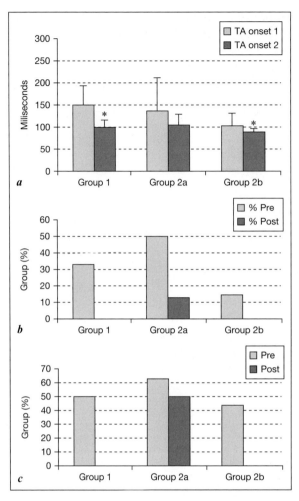

Fig. 1. Group 1 received TC only (TC). The control group first received control training (2a). After post-control training testing they then received TC (2b). ***a*** TA onset latency is shown for each group. Onset 1 indicates before the intervention and onset 2 after the intervention. ***b, c*** Groups 1 and 2b do not have a post-intervention bar because they eliminated reversed activation (i.e. GA onset before TA) and cocontraction. Reprinted with permission from Gatts and Woollacott [9].

295 ms longer to activate their GA after TC training. GA muscle burst duration was significantly reduced in group 1, although controls approached significance (p ≤ 0.060). After TC, controls further reduced their GA duration for a total reduction in GA burst duration of 178.61 ms. The lack of

significance in group 2b was probably due to a threshold in the total reduction possible relative to the task. After training, both the TC and control groups improved their muscle response organization by activating the TA before the GA. This is a functionally appropriate response employed to help reposition a lagging center of mass forward toward the right leg that was rapidly moved forward by the platform acceleration. Figure 1b illustrates that all groups reduced occurrence of reversed activation after the training, although not significantly. Odds of reversed activation occurring after training was almost identical after both interventions: (6.23 times less occurrence after TC versus 6.16 times less after control training). However, only TC eliminated reversed activation.

Figure 1c illustrates pre-post changes in cocontraction during recovery. Only TC group 1 changed significantly (p ≤ 0.016). Note that TC group 2b also eliminated cocontraction. Combining both TC groups to examine effects of training, we found odds of a cocontraction occurring was significantly less after TC training [TC = 18 times less compared to 1.6 times less after control training (TC 18:1, p ≤ 0.003, control 1.6:1, p ≤ 1.0)]. This means TC was highly effective in reducing TA and GA coactivation during a large/fast perturbation delivered while walking in balance-impaired seniors. This is important because coactivation reflects increased expenditure of energy used to regain balance and lengthens the time for restoring joint/segment angular trajectories used to maintain the gait cycle [8]. Thus, if this response were eliminated, balance responses would likely be faster. This conclusion was supported by our EMG data (table 3, fig. 1a, c).

Figure 2 presents pre- and post-TC training EMG data from an 86-year-old subject at high risk for falling. Before starting the TC training, she had fallen 3 times and could not get up. Figure 2a illustrates both a reversed activation and coactivation of the GA and TA muscles. This response disrupted the gait cycle and required the subject to drop the left swing leg to the ground to prevent falling backward. Post-TC training (fig. 2b) shows improved muscle activation characteristics associated with smooth recovery and continuation of the gait cycle. The TA is activated before the GA, there is no coactivation, muscle bursts are clearly defined and maintain the on/off coordination of a healthy gait cycle. Notice the voltage produced by the GA has increased fourfold after TC balance training.

The percent of time a muscle was active from heelstrike to toeoff is shown in table 3 as %TA or %GA duration. None of the groups changed significantly in %TA duration. The crossover group's (i.e. control = 2a, TC = 2b) %GA duration was not significantly different but the duration in group 1 was significantly reduced following TC (p ≤ 0.012). The decline was likely related to a significant reduction in GA burst duration in group 1.

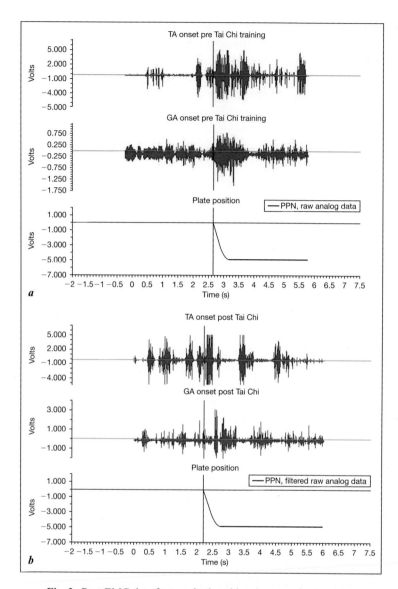

Fig. 2. Raw EMG data from a single subject in group 1. Plate onset is indicated by the vertical line. *a* Muscular activation problems are shown by the GA onset occurring before the TA onset and both muscles are cocontracting the entire time the plate is moving. This caused the subject to drop the swing leg to the ground to prevent a fall. *b* After TC (TC) training muscle characteristics improve. TA onset occurs before the GA and cocontraction is eliminated. Muscles' bursts are clearly defined and maintain the on/off coordination of a healthy gait cycle. Note the fourfold increase in GA voltage after TC training. Reprinted with permission from Gatts and Woollacott [9].

Discussion

Prior research found older adults had difficulty maintaining a normal gait cycle during recovery from a slip due to delayed distal muscle activation, high rates of cocontraction, and prolonged muscle bursts [8]. These responses resulted in a decreased forward momentum, backward fall of the trunk, interruption of the gait cycle, and dropping the swing leg to the ground in order to regain balance. In the present study, we examined the effect of TC and control training on neuromuscular mechanisms controlling the ankle joint of the perturbed leg during large/fast forward movement of the base of support during walking. Responses from the TA are important because previous work found responses serve to resist change in rotation of the perturbed ankle joint during gait progression and help speed up the body's rate of forward progression to realign the whole body center of mass over the perturbed stance leg [30]. GA responses are important because they strongly respond to ankle joint displacement and can prevent the shank from efficiently rolling over the foot, which acts to impede the continuation of gait [31]. Overall, responses from muscles controlling the ankle joint are significant elicitors for reactive postural responses in perturbed gait. We also examined four commonly used clinical balance measures in order to see if similar trends existed between lab and clinical measures of balance improvement because these clinical tests have been shown to correlate with functional mobility [13, 32].

All clinical measures significantly improved in TC group 1 while five of six measures improved significantly for crossover TC group 2b. Control training (group 2a) improved significantly only on FR, and after TC the same subjects reached 4.22 inches further ($p \leq 0.0002$). Thus, the TC balance training not only affected the lower body, it also transferred to significant increase in limits of stability in the forward region and range of motion in the axial spinal column. EMG results indicated neuromuscular mechanisms supporting balance control demonstrated a similar trend to clinical measures. Only TC training significantly reduced TA response time (group 1, $p \leq 0.004$; group 2b, $p \leq 0.028$) and the occurrence of a cocontraction ($p \leq 0.003$) of the agonist and antagonist muscles. This supported our hypothesis. After TC, the TA activated up to 50 ms faster. This is worthy of note because the TC intervention used slow movements, yet the effect of training transferred to significantly faster muscle onset in both TC trained groups. This may be related to the elimination of cocontraction in TC-trained groups. Reduction or elimination of cocontraction keeps the muscles and joints flexible. This would allow muscles to respond more quickly while making adjustments required to restore a disrupted base of support, help restore forward momentum and continue the gait cycle. Control training did not significantly reduce either TA onset time or cocontraction rates. However, TC and control training were very similar in their ability to reduce the occurrence of reversed activation.

Previous research examining muscle response onsets in unstable versus healthy seniors found similar onset latency differences to the pre-TC versus post-TC improvements we found in our study [33]. Interestingly, after the TC intervention improvements made by balance-impaired subjects in our study were larger. These results indicated that older adults with functional balance problems have slower onset latencies and those who are functionally well balanced show latencies within our range from pre- to post-training.

Berger et al. [28] suggested the early part of an EMG signal from leg muscles during stumbling represented complex reactions generated in a spinal pathway by group II and III afferents and were probably controlled by supraspinal centers. Our results showed TC training improved reactive postural responses in neural mechanisms controlling the ankle joint of the perturbed stance leg. Thus, changes in responses we found may involve a key polysynaptic spinal or brainstem reflex loop involved with dynamic balance responses because such responses have been shown to react within 70–90 ms of perturbation in healthy young adults. This onset is faster than vestibular or visually mediated activation, and these responses can be modified by training and experience [8, 28, 34].

Rapid, correct, and plastic neuromuscular activation is crucial for controlling the high-speed task-specific, yet quickly changing dynamics required to prevent a fall. The central nervous system must select the correct muscles for the task. These muscles must be activated and inhibited in the proper sequence and relationship, at the appropriate time, force, and duration. A series of linked events sets up a 'domino effect' if the neuromuscular activation and coordination is inappropriate. For example, if the TA of the weight-bearing leg delays activation to a forward slip of its foot, the body's center of mass lags dangerously behind the forward moving base of support. If a reversed activation occurs, a GA contraction contributes to further backward falling. This event necessitates the contralateral leg interrupt its forward swing by dropping to the ground to create a new base of support. This backward movement interrupts the gait cycle and requires additional and appropriate control of muscle forces, segmental coordination and anatomical positioning. Lastly, the central nervous system must initiate a new gait cycle.

Both interventions were similar in their ability to improve muscle activation sequencing (6.23 times less reversed activation after TC versus controls 6.16). Only TC eliminated cocontraction and reversed activation and improved TA onset by up to 50 ms. Clinical measures demonstrated a similar trend; TC groups improved significantly on more measures than did controls. Thus, the TC intervention transferred to improvements on four measures of functional balance efficacy. Kinematic and force plate data collected simultaneously with our EMG data supported this conclusion: TC training was associated with significantly reduced compensatory backward stepping ($p \leq 0.003$), significantly more efficient recovery step positioning used to continue gait ($p \leq 0.001$) and significantly improved control of recovery step width ($p \leq 0.034$), while controls showed no significant change [10].

How might the TC protocol we used have contributed to our results? Although traditional TC training incorporates educational factors regarding posture and balance control, relating movement performance to fall prevention strategies was a significant departure from TC interventions previously reported in clinical journals. As in traditional TC training, we regard the cognitive element as an important factor to enhance and internalize the new motor skills. One of the differences between our study and previous studies [1, 35] that may have led to strong training effects was that we concentrated on TC movement principles within each single form rather than linking postures into sequences. Lastly, our training was both shorter (3 weeks) and more intense than most others, with sessions 5 days/week for 1.5 h/day.

We did not measure bilateral muscles of the ankle, knee and trunk because previous research [8] indicated seniors had equivalent slowing of muscular responses in both the ipsilateral and the contralateral leg when compared to young adults. The muscles we chose as representing the 10 muscles Tang and Woollacott used were the TA (activated first) and its antagonist, because slowing of the TA was representative of other agonist muscles of the ipsi- and contralateral legs and the GA responses were representative of antagonist cocontraction that tended to be observed at other joints as well as the ankle joint. This characterization of responses at the ankle joint allowed us to analyze fewer variables, yet gather key information about improvements in response characteristics associated with TC training [9, 10].

Complimentary and alternative medical practices are increasingly utilized by the general population. However, how these practices achieve their beneficial effects is still largely unclear. Data from our study help clarify how neural mechanisms can benefit from TC training. The likelihood that TC training would transfer to balance improvement in the real world was also supported by significant improvements on four widely used and validated clinical tests of functional balance [13, 30]: TUG, Single leg stance time, Tandem stance time, and FR (table 2). Overall, TC training significantly reduced neuromuscular response time, enhanced flexibility in the ankle joint by significantly reducing cocontraction, and improved functional coordination of agonist-antagonist activation in muscles controlling the ankle of the perturbed single stance leg during recovery of balance. TC also significantly improved the ability to control stepping strategies and continue the gait cycle [10].

Current evidence indicates TC balance recovery principles may be combined with mechanical training aids to reduce trip-related falls in older women.

We recently applied our TC experience training older adults to the design and implementation of task-specific, individualized training protocols incorporating an obstacle and computerized treadmill. Current data from the ongoing study indicate motor skills acquired on the treadmill transfer to walking overground. In response to an unexpected trip during overground walking, the fall rate of untrained controls was 22.6% compared to zero for trained subjects, and the treadmill-acquired motor skills were retained for 1 month [36].

Overall, our results can be used to (a) guide clinicians interested in 'evidence-based practice', (b) support TC's acceptance by medical communities, and (c) promote referrals for TC as a neuromuscular balance rehabilitation therapy.

References

1   Wolf S, Barnhart H, Kutner N, et al: Reducing frailty and falls in older persons: an investigation of Tai Chi and computerized balance training. J Am Geriatr Soc 1996;44:489–497.
2   Wolfson L, Whipple R, Derby C, et al: Balance and strength training in older adults: Intervention gains and Tai Chi maintenance. J Am Geriatr Soc 1996;44:498–506.
3   Yan J: Tai Chi practice improves senior citizens' balance and arm movement control. J Aging Phys Act 1998;6:271–284.
4   Thornton EW, Sykes KS, Tang Wk: Health benefits of Tai Chi exercise: improved balance and blood pressure in middle-aged women. Health Promot Int 2004;19:33–38.
5   Tsang WW, Wong VS, Fu SN, Hui-Chan CW: Tai Chi improves standing balance control under reduced or conflicting sensory conditions. Arch Phys Med Rehabil 2004;85:129–137.
6   Wang C, Collet J, Lau J: The effect of Tai Chi on health outcomes in patients with chronic conditions. Arch Intern Med 2004;164:493–501.
7   Ellis A, Trent R: Do the risks and consequences of hospitalized fall injuries among older adults in California vary by type of fall? J Gerontol A Biol Sci Med Sci 2001;56A:M686–M692.
8   Tang P, Woollacott M: Inefficient postural responses to unexpected slips during walking in older adults. J Gerontol 1998;53A:M471–M480.
9   Gatts SK, Woollacott MH: Neural mechanisms underlying balance improvement with short term Tai Chi training. Aging Clin Exp Res 2006;18:7–19.
10 Gatts SK, Woollacott MH: How Tai Chi improves balance: Biomechanics of recovery to a walking slip in impaired seniors. Gait Posture 2007;25:205–214. Epub 2006 May 2.
11 Duncan P, Studenski S, Chandler J, Prescott B: Functional reach: a new clinical measure of balance. J Gerontol 1990;45:M192–M197.
12 Podsiadlo D, Richardson S: The timed 'Up and Go' test: a test of basic functional mobility for frail elderly persons. J Am Geriatr Soc 1991;39:142–148.
13 Woollacott M, Shumway-Cook A: Clinical and research methodology for the study of posture and balance; in Masdeu J, et al (eds): Gait Disorders of Aging. Philadelphia: Lippincott-Raven, 1997, pp 107–121.
14 Shumway-Cook A, Woollacott M: Clinical management of the patient with a postural control disorder. Motor Control. Baltimore: Lippincott Williams & Wilkins, 2001, p 273.
15 Schenkman M, Morey M, Kuchibhatla M: Spinal flexibility and balance control among community-dwelling adults with and without Parkinson disease. J Gerontol 2000;55:441–445.
16 Mahoney R, Barthel D: Functional evaluation: The Barthel Index. Maryland Med J 1965;14:61–65.
17 Wolfson L: Balance decrements in older persons: Effects of age and disease; in Masdeu J, et al (eds): Gait Disorders of Aging. Philadelphia: Lippincott-Raven, 1997, pp 79–91.
18 Bogle Thorbahn L, Newton R: Use of the Berg balance test to predict falls in elderly persons. Phys Ther 1996;76:576–585.

19 Fu Z: Mastering Yang style taijiquan. (translation by Swain L). Berkeley: North Atlantic Books, 1999, pp 12–13.
20 Ho'o M: Health benefits of the form. Tai Chi Chuan: The 27 Forms. Burbank: Ohara Publications Inc., 1986, pp109–111.
21 Whipple, R: Improving balance in older adults: Identifying the significant training stimuli; in Masdeu J, et al (eds): Gait Disorders of Aging. Philadelphia: Lippincott-Raven, 1997, pp 355–379.
22 Elbe R: Changes in gait with normal aging; in Masdeu J, et al (eds): Gait Disorders of Aging. Philadelphia: Lippincott-Raven, 1997, pp 93–105.
23 Northwest physical therapy services. Safety and gait enhancement. Seattle, WA 98133.
24 Tideikasaar R: Environmental factors in the prevention of falls; in Masdeu J, et al (eds): Gait Disorders of Aging. Philadelphia: Lippincott-Raven, 1997, pp 395–412.
25 Schenkman M: The Axial mobility program; in Masdeu J, et al (eds): Gait Disorders of Aging. Philadelphia: Lippincott-Raven, 1997, pp 415–427.
26 Friedrich J: Tension control techniques to combat stress; in Harris R, Frankel J (eds): Guide to Fitness after Fifty. New York: Plenum Press, 1977, pp 323–336.
27 Nashner L: Physiology of balance, with special reference to the healthy elderly; in Masdeu J, et al (eds): Gait Disorders of Aging. Philadelphia: Lippincott-Raven, 1997, pp 37–53.
28 Berger W, Dietz V, Quintern J: Corrective reactions to stumbling in man: neuronal co-ordination of bilateral leg muscle activity during gait. J Physiol 1984;357:109–25.
29 Strandberg L, Lanshammar H: On the biomechanics of slipping accidents; in Matsui H, Kobayashi K (eds): Biomechanics VIII-A. (International series on biomechanics, Vol 4A). Champaign: Human Kinetics Publishers, 1981, pp 397–402.
30 Nashner L: Balance adjustments of humans perturbed while walking. J Neurophysiol 1980;44: 650–664.
31 Stein R: Reflex modulation during locomotion: functional significance; in Patla A (ed): Adaptability of Human Gait. Amsterdam, the Netherlands: Elsevier Science Publishers BV, 1991, pp 21–36.
32 Berg K, Wood-Dauphinee S, Williams J: Measuring balance in the elderly: validation of an instrument. Can J Public Health 1992;83:S9–S11.
33 Lin S, Woollacott M: Postural muscle responses following changing balance threats in young, stable older and unstable older adults. J Motor Behav 2002;34:37–44.
34 Horak F, Nashner L: Central programming of postural movements: adaptation to altered support surface configurations. J Neurophysiol 1986;55:1369–1381.
35 Wolf S, Sattin R, Kutner M, et al: Intense Tai Chi exercise training and fall occurrences in older, transitionally frail adults: A randomized, controlled trial. J Am Geriatr Soc 2003;51:1693–1701.
36 Gatts SK, et al: Older women reduce falls due to a trip after task-specific training. In preparation.

Strawberry Gatts, PhD
Clinical Biomechanics and Rehabilitation Lab., Department of Kinesiology
University of Illinois at Chicago College of Applied Health Sciences
1919 W. Taylor St., Chicago, IL 60612 (USA)
Tel. +1 312 413 7762, Fax +1 312 996 3532
E-Mail sgatts@uic.edu, sgatts@uoneuro.uoregon.edu, sgatts@hotmail.com

Hong Y (ed): Tai Chi Chuan. State of the Art in International Research.
Med Sport Sci. Basel, Karger, 2008, vol 52, pp 104–114

....

Sensorimotor Control of Balance: A Tai Chi Solution for Balance Disorders in Older Subjects

William W.N. Tsang, Christina W.Y. Hui-Chan

Department of Rehabilitation Sciences, The Hong Kong Polytechnic University, Hong Kong, SAR, China

Abstract

Background/Aims: In addition to environmental factors, deteriorating sensorimotor control of balance will predispose older adults to falls. Understanding the aging effects on sensorimotor control of balance performance is important for designing fall prevention programs for older adults. How repeated practice of Tai Chi can improve limb joint proprioception, integration of neural signals in the central nervous system for balance control, and motor output at the level of knee muscles is discussed in this chapter. **Results:** Our previous studies showed that elderly Tai Chi practitioners performed significantly better than elderly nonpractitioners in (1) knee joint proprioception, (2) reduced or conflicting sensory situations that demand more visual or vestibular contributions, (3) standing balance control after vestibular stimulation without visual input, (4) voluntary weight shifting in different directions within the base of support, (5) single-leg stance during perturbations of the support surface, and (6) knee extensor and flexor muscle strength. In a prospective study, we further showed that 4 weeks of daily Tai Chi practice but not general education produced significant improvement in balance performance. **Conclusion:** The requirements of Tai Chi for accurate joint positioning and weight transfer involving smooth coordination of neck, trunk, upper and lower limb movements, make it particularly useful for improving the sensorimotor control of balance in the elderly. Because Tai Chi can be practiced any time and anywhere, and is well accepted by older people in both the East and now the West, it is especially suited to be a key component of a low-costing community-based fall prevention program alongside with education about environmental factors.

The world population is aging. The number of people aged 90–99 years is expected to rise from just over 8 million in 2002 to 60 million in 2050 [1]. Falls have been identified as one of the major causes of morbidity and mortality in

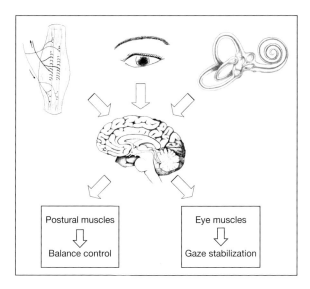

Fig. 1. Sensorimotor control of balance.

older adults [2]. Approximately 32% of community-dwelling elderly over the age of 75 fall at least once a year [3]. In the United States, the cost of hip fractures in the elderly attributed to falls has been reported to be about USD 10 billion in 2001 [4]. This represents a major financial burden for society.

In addition to environmental factors, physiological factors intrinsic to older adults are known to predispose them to falls [5–7]. It is therefore important to understand the effects of aging on the control of balance when designing fall prevention programs for older people.

Sensorimotor control of balance is complex (fig. 1). On the input side, 3 sensory systems are involved. These are: somatosensory, visual and vestibular systems. They contribute to the coordination of the axial (neck and trunk) and limb muscles against gravity to different degrees depending on the environmental conditions. To achieve appropriate balance control, all the relevant information from the 3 sensory systems will first be integrated by the central nervous system (CNS) [8]. Control of the position of head and body in space then requires the generation and coordination of appropriate muscle forces by descending pathways to counteract gravity in such a way as to maintain the head and body in equilibrium over the base of support. However, both sensory systems (input) and muscle strength (output) are known to deteriorate with age. When degeneration is severe, it could affect balance control and predispose these older subjects to falls [5, 9, 10]. In this article, we will first discuss the problems arising from sensorimotor control of balance due to aging, namely the 3 sensory systems, integration of sensorimotor signals in the CNS, and motor output via limb muscles, then review the effects of Tai Chi on these components of balance control.

Sensory Input: Limb Proprioception

Limb proprioception is a sense of the 'position' and 'movement' of one's own limbs in the absence of vision, termed 'limb position sense' and 'kinesthesia', respectively [8]. Limb proprioception has been found to diminish with age, after ligamentous injuries, and as a result of some pathological conditions such as stroke and osteoarthritis [11, 12]. More importantly, older fallers have been shown to have significantly reduced proprioception of their lower limbs [13, 14].

Tai Chi puts great emphasis on exact joint positioning and the direction of limb movement. Therefore, we hypothesized that repeated practice of Tai Chi would develop a heightened sense of limb joint position in Tai Chi practitioners. To focus on joint proprioceptive input without motor involvement, we developed a passive joint repositioning paradigm for testing knee joint position sense with excellent repeatability (ICC = 0.90) [15]. In that study, elderly Tai Chi practitioners and control subjects similar in age, gender and physical activity level were compared in terms of the acuity of their knee joint proprioception. Tai Chi practitioners with a mean of 10.1 (SD 9.5) years of experience were shown to have better knee joint proprioceptive acuity (average absolute angle error = $2.1 \pm 1.2°$) when compared with that of control subjects ($4.0 \pm 3.4°$, p = 0.023) [15]. Better joint proprioception in Tai Chi practitioners has also been found by other investigators when the 'threshold' for detecting joint movement test was measured at the knee and ankle joints [16], and in an active joint repositioning test at the knee [17]. Our study further showed that absolute angle error in the knee joint repositioning test had a significantly positive correlation with reaction time (r = 0.572, p = 0.000) and a significantly negative correlation with the maximum excursion of the center of gravity (r = -0.340, p = 0.034) during subject's voluntary weight shifting to different spatial limits of stability, in the so-called 'limits of stability test' [15, 18]. These results highlighted the importance of knee joint position sense in functional activities involving leaning or weight shifting during upright stance.

Drawing from the knowledge garnered from contemporary neuroimaging studies, we purported that improved joint proprioception as a result of long-term Tai Chi practice could have induced plastic changes in the cortex [15]. Tai Chi practice requiring repeated precise positioning of body and limb joints in space could bring about increased discharges of the muscle spindle receptors

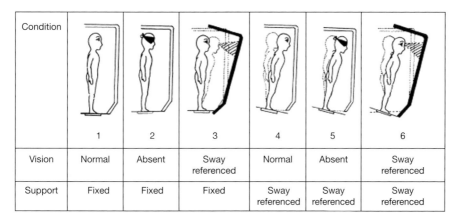

Condition	1	2	3	4	5	6
Vision	Normal	Absent	Sway referenced	Normal	Absent	Sway referenced
Support	Fixed	Fixed	Fixed	Sway referenced	Sway referenced	Sway referenced

Fig. 2. Sensory organization test for 6 different sensory conditions.

through descending commands via α-γ co-activation during voluntary movements and increased output of the appropriate muscles [19]. Findings from neuroimaging studies suggested that the resultant increased afferent input and efferent output would increase the strength of synaptic connections in the involved pathways and/or afferent-induced plastic (structural) changes in the brain [20, 21].

However, these findings on lower limb joint proprioception were obtained in studies with cross-sectional designs, so a causal relationship between Tai Chi practice and improved joint proprioception has yet to be examined through a prospective intervention study.

Integration of Sensorimotor Signals in the CNS for Proper Balance Control

Depending on the environmental context under which proper balance control is required, Nashner [22] suggested that the weighting given to a sensory modality providing less accurate information will be reduced, while the weighting of sensory modalities providing more accurate information will be increased. He termed the process of selecting and integrating appropriate sensory information at the level of the CNS 'sensory organization' (fig. 2) [22]. The inability to select and integrate appropriate sensory information to produce appropriate balance responses may be another factor which predisposes the elderly subjects to fall. Wallmann [23] compared elderly fallers with nonfallers and found that fallers swayed significantly more when the supporting platform swayed in the same direction and magnitude of the subjects.

Balance Control under Reduced or Conflicting Sensory Conditions

Practicing Tai Chi involves head-and-body and limb movements which would stimulate the somatosensory, visual and vestibular systems. The question of whether long-term, repeated Tai Chi practice can improve balance control in the presence of reduced or conflicting somatosensory, visual and vestibular conditions had been addressed by our research group [24] and by Wong et al. [25]. We tested subjects under 6 combinations of sensory conditions: with their eyes open, eyes closed, or sway-referenced visual surround, and with the supporting surface fixed or sway referenced (fig. 2). Our findings showed that elderly Tai Chi practitioners exhibited better balance control when they stood under conditions that demanded an increased reliance on the visual and vestibular systems than nonpractitioners similar in age, gender, and physical activity level [24]. Of particular interest is that these older Tai Chi practitioners even attained a level of balance control performance similar to that of young, healthy subjects, especially when there was an increased reliance on the visual and vestibular systems [26]. Wong et al. [25] also showed that Tai Chi practitioners swayed significantly less than did a control group in the more challenging condition where the somatosensory input was off-set by absent or conflicting visual input.

Balance Control after Excessive Vestibular Stimulation

Somatosensory cues from the support surface and visual cues from the external environment can provide adequate information to maintain balance control only when they can serve as correct references, such as when the support surface or the visual surround is fixed. The vestibular system provides information about the position and movement of the head with respect to gravity and to inertial forces. Thus, it is not similarly influenced by changes in surface and visual conditions. Vestibular input can provide a reference that could be invoked to suppress conflicting somatosensory and visual inputs. However, degeneration of the vestibular receptor with aging [27] can mean that some elderly persons can no longer rely on adequate or accurate vestibular input to maintain their balance.

After whole head-and-body rotation, a subject has to suppress erroneous hyperactive postrotational vestibular cues and rely on properly weighted somatosensory input to maintain normal standing balance. Figure 3 shows a representative subject sitting on a rotational chair with her head fixed at 30° angle below the horizontal plane so as to selectively stimulate her horizontal semicircular canals [28]. After whole head-and-body rotation at 80°/s for 60 s

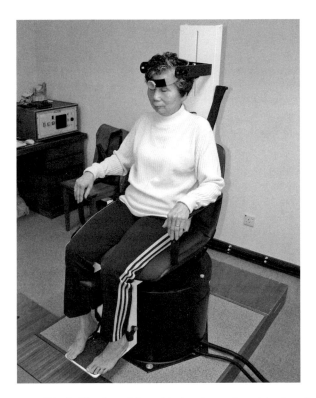

Fig. 3. Fixation of the subject and experimental set-up for whole head-and-body rotation using a rotational chair.

with eyes closed, she was told to stand up immediately with her eyes still closed. In order to maintain quiet standing without undue sway, subjects must suppress erroneous vestibular inputs by relying on correct somatosensory inputs in the absence of visual input.

Our results showed that elderly subjects exhibited significantly within-group increases in anteroposterior (AP) and mediolateral sway after vestibular stimulation ($p < 0.001$ for all measures), but Tai Chi practitioners of similar age exhibited less sway in the AP direction. Furthermore, significantly smaller percentage increases in total sway path, peak amplitude and mean velocity of body sway in the AP direction were found in Tai Chi practitioners when compared with those of control subjects ($p = 0.003–0.016$) [28]. Significantly better performance in the Tai Chi practitioners could be the result of improvements in joint proprioception [15–17], central integration [26, 29], and/or muscle strength [30]. Whatever the mechanism, the improved balance control should help older adults to better maintain their balance even when they are subject to

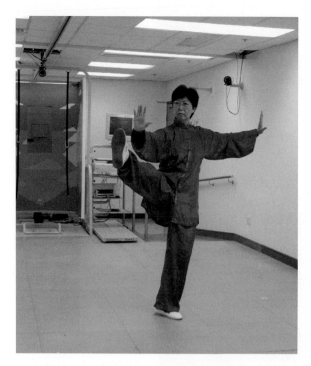

Fig. 4. The 'kick with the heel' maneuver.

excessive vestibular stimulation. Thus, Tai Chi could be an effective component of a fall prevention program for older persons even when they face more challenging situations requiring proper balance control.

Balance Control during Weight Shifting and Perturbed Single-Leg Stance
Impaired balance performance has been identified as a major factor that causes falls in the elderly [5]. Tai Chi practice involves precisely controlled weight transfer during voluntary shifts of the body in double-leg stance, and from double- to single-leg stance, as exemplified by a Tai Chi form called 'kick with the heel' maneuver (fig. 4). Will these practitioners be able to control their limits of stability better than their healthy counterparts? Results from our study showed that elderly Tai Chi practitioners initiated voluntary shifting of their weight to different spatial positions within their base of support more quickly (reaction time, p = 0.008), leaned their body further without losing their stability (maximum excursion, p = 0.001), and showed better control of their leaning trajectory than control subjects (p = 0.008) [15]. However, it is well known that

falls seldom occur during double-leg stance, as the centre of mass is well within the base of support [9]. We therefore examined the control of body sway in single-leg stance on a support surface being perturbed by forward or backward platform movement [30]. Our findings demonstrated that Tai Chi practitioners manifested smaller AP body sway angles in perturbed single-leg stance than did control subjects (p < 0.001).

Lower Limb Muscle Strength and Balance Control

Muscle size and related neuromuscular function are known to decrease with age. The decline in muscle strength is largely not discerned until about the sixth decade of life [31]. Patla et al. [32] compared healthy elderly subjects (mean age = 69 years) with young subjects (mean age = 20 years) by asking them to step forward, sideways or backward with a designated leg in response to a light signal. Analysis of the vertical force component of the movements revealed that elderly subjects took longer to reach peak force in all 3 stepping directions, and they produced lower peak force during forward stepping. Note that the peak force developed in the stepping leg was required to transfer body weight to the nonstepping leg. These findings strongly suggested that the muscles of the elderly subjects were weaker from a functional perspective than those of young persons. Such deficits could play a role in impaired postural control, resulting in falls among the elderly [4, 33].

To address possible effects of Tai Chi practice on muscle strength, we compared concentric and eccentric isokinetic test results of dominant knee flexors and extensors at an angular velocity of 30°/s between Tai Chi practitioners and control subjects similar in age, gender and activity level [30]. Our results showed that elderly Tai Chi practitioners had significantly greater peak torque–body weight ratio in concentric and eccentric isokinetic contractions of knee flexor and extensor muscles (p < 0.05). Moreover, the extent of strength increase was similar between knee extensors and knee flexors. These findings differed from those of Wu et al. [34], who found no difference in knee flexor strength between Tai Chi practitioners and the control group when isokinetic evaluation of their Tai Chi practitioners was conducted at 60 and 120°/s. Our study [30] adopted a slower isokinetic testing speed, as Tai Chi involves mainly slow movements, and this training specificity may explain our finding of stronger knee flexors besides knee extensors among the Tai Chi practitioners. The results further showed that knee muscle strength in the elderly was negatively correlated with body sway angles in AP perturbed single-leg stance (r = −0.335 to −0.529, p < 0.05 or 0.01). These findings again highlighted the importance of knee muscle strength in actual balance performance.

Tai Chi as a Fall Prevention Program

From a practical point of view, older subjects may not have the time or wish to spend a long time to learn a fall prevention program. So, the question arises as to how long will an elderly subject need to practice Tai Chi to achieve significant improvements in sensorimotor control of balance? We conducted a prospective study with older subjects similar in age, gender, height and weight who voluntarily participated in either supervised Tai Chi or general education for 1.5 h a day, 6 times a week, for 8 weeks [29]. This randomized control trial showed that 4 weeks of daily Tai Chi practice was sufficient to produce significant improvements in the sensorimotor control of balance performance in older subjects, as measured by significantly less body sway when standing under conditions requiring an increased reliance on the vestibular system ($p = 0.006$) and better directional control in the limits of stability test ($p = 0.018$), when compared with those of the control group receiving general education. Of importance is that the gains in these novice Tai Chi practitioners were comparable to those of experienced practitioners with 7–10 years of Tai Chi, and were maintained even at 4 weeks after the intervention ended.

Conclusion

Degeneration of the sensory and motor systems involved with balance control in the older adults due to aging could be substantial. How Tai Chi improves each component of the sensorimotor control of balance has been presented in the studies reviewed above. Briefly, studies from our research group and others have shown that repeated practice of Tai Chi improved the practitioners' joint proprioception, integration of sensorimotor signals in the CNS, knee muscle strength, and balance control under more challenging conditions. The latter could be reduced/conflicting sensory conditions after excessive vestibular stimulation, intentional weight shifting within the base of support and/or single-leg support on a moving platform. Because Tai Chi can be practiced by older adults any time and anywhere, it is particularly suited to preventing or slowing down the development of balance disorders in this age group. In fact, Tai Chi practice has already been shown to be effective in helping to prevent falls among older adults [35, 36]. In contrast to Western exercises requiring exercise equipment and/or a gymnasium, Tai Chi is relatively low costing. Once learned, it could be practiced any time and anywhere, in parks or any outdoor or indoor space in hospitals, community center or even at home. Therefore, municipal governments should widely promote the teaching of Tai Chi in the parks and through community and old age centers.

References

1   Kalache A, Aboderin I, Hoskins I: Compression of morbidity and active ageing: Key priorities for public health policy in the 21st century. Bull World Health Org 2002;80:243–244.
2   Tinetti ME: Preventing falls in elderly persons. New Engl J Med 2003;348:42–49.
3   Tinetti ME, Speechley M, Ginter SF: Risk factors for falls among elderly persons living in the community. New Engl J Med 1988;319:1701–1707.
4   Carter ND, Kannus P, Khan KM: Exercise in the prevention of falls in older people: A systematic literature review examining the rationale and the evidence. Sports Med 2001;31:427–438.
5   Berg KO, Kairy D: Balance interventions to prevent falls. Generations 2002;26:75–78.
6   Lin SI, Woollacott MH: Postural muscle responses following changing balance threats in young, stable older, and unstable older adults. J Mot Behav 2002;34:37–44.
7   Shumway-Cook A, Brauer S, Woollacott M: Predicting the probability for falls in community-dwelling older adults using the Timed Up & Go Test. Phys Ther 2000;80:896–903.
8   Gardner ER, Martin JH, Jessell TM: The bodily senses; in Kandel ER, Schwartz JH, Jessell TM (eds): Principles of Neural Science. New York, McGraw-Hill, 2000, pp 430–449.
9   Clark S, Rose DJ: Evaluation of dynamic balance among community-dwelling older adult fallers: A generalizability study of the limits of stability test. Arch Phys Med Rehabil 2001;82:468–474.
10   Patla A, Frank J, Winter D: Assessment of balance control in the elderly: Major issues. Physiother Can 1990;42:89–97.
11   Skinner HB, Barrack RL, Cook SD: Age-related declines in proprioception. Clin Orthop Relat R 1984;184:208–211.
12   Yan T, Hui-Chan CWY: Ability to detect movement of the knee joint decreases with age. Arch Phys Med Rehabil 2000;81:1274.
13   Lord SR, Rogers MW, Howland A, Fitzpatrick R: Lateral stability, sensorimotor function and falls in older people. J Am Geriatr Soc 1999;47:1077–1081.
14   Sorock GS, Labiner DM: Peripheral neuromuscular dysfunction and falls in an elderly cohort. Am J Epidemiol 1992;136:584–591.
15   Tsang WWN, Hui-Chan CWY: Effects of Tai Chi on joint proprioception and stability limits in elderly subjects. Med Sci Sports Exerc 2003;35:1962–1971.
16   Xu D, Hong Y, Li J, Chan K: Effect of tai chi exercise on proprioception of ankle and knee joints in old people. Br J Sports Med 2004;38:50–54.
17   Fong SM, Ng GY: The effects of sensorimotor performance and balance with Tai Chi training. Arch Phys Med Rehabil 2006;87:82–87.
18   Tsang WWN, Hui-Chan CWY: Effects of exercise on joint sense and balance in elderly men: Tai Chi versus golf. Med Sci Sports Exerc 2004;36:658–667.
19   Kandel ER, Schwartz JH, Jessell TM: Principles of Neural Science. New York, McGraw-Hill, 2000.
20   Rossini PM, Calautti C, Pauri F, Baron JC: Post-stroke plastic reorganization in the adult brain. Lancet Neurol 2003;2:493–502.
21   Schaechter JD: Motor rehabilitation and brain plasticity after hemiparetic stroke. Prog Neurobiol 2004;73:61–72.
22   Nashner LM: Evaluation of postural stability, movement and control; in Hasson SM (eds): Clinical Exercise Physiology. St. Louis, Mosby, 1994, pp 199–234.
23   Wallmann HW: Comparison of elderly nonfallers and fallers on performance measures of functional reach, sensory organization, and limits of stability. J Gerontol Ser A Biol Sci Med Sci 2001;56:M580–M583.
24   Tsang WWN, Wong V, Hui-Chan CWY: A comparison of balance control under different sensory conditions between elderly Tai Chi and non-Tai Chi practitioners; in Duysens J, Smits-Engelsman BCM, Kingma H (eds): Control of Posture and Gait. Maastricht, Netherlands: International Society for Postural and Gait Research, 2001, pp 382–387.
25   Wong AM, Lin YC, Chou SW, Tang FT, Wong PY: Coordination exercise and postural stability in elderly people: Effect of Tai Chi Chuan. Arch Phys Med Rehabil 2001;82:608–612.
26   Tsang WW, Wong VS, Fu SN, Hui-Chan CW: Tai Chi improves standing balance control under reduced or conflicting sensory conditions. Arch Phys Med Rehabil 2004;85:129–137.

27 Rosenhall U, Rubin W: Degenerative changes in the human vestibular sensory epithelia. Acta Otolaryngol (Stockh) 1975;79:67–80.
28 Tsang WWN, Hui-Chan CWY: Standing balance after vestibular stimulation in Tai Chi-practicing and nonpracticing healthy older adults. Arch Phys Med Rehabil 2006;87:546–553.
29 Tsang WWN, Hui-Chan CWY: Effect of 4- and 8-wk intensive Tai Chi training on balance control in the elderly. Med Sci Sports Exerc 2004;36:648–657.
30 Tsang WWN, Hui-Chan CWY: Comparison of muscle torque, balance, and confidence in older Tai Chi and healthy adults. Med Sci Sports Exerc 2005;37:280–289.
31 Vandervoort AA: Aging of the human neuromuscular system. Muscle Nerve 2002;25:17–25.
32 Patla AE, Frank JS, Winter DA, Rietdyk S, Prentice S, Prasad S: Age-related changes in balance control system: Initiation of stepping. Clin Biomech 1993;8:179–184.
33 Schwendner KI, Mikesky AE, Holt WS Jr, Peacock M, Burr DB: Differences in muscle endurance and recovery between fallers and nonfallers, and between young and older women. J Gerontol 1997;52:M155–M160.
34 Wu G, Zhao F, Zhou X, Liu W: Improvement of isokinetic knee extensor strength and reduction of postural sway in the elderly from long-term Tai Chi exercise. Arch Phys Med Rehabil 2002;83: 1364–1369.
35 Wolf SL, Barnhart HX, Kutner NG, McNeely E, Coogler C, Xu T: Reducing frailty and falls in older persons: An investigation of Tai Chi and computerized balance training. J Am Geriatr Soc 1996;44:487–497.
36 Li F, Harmer P, Fisher KJ, McAuley E, Chaumeton N, Eckstrom E, Wilson NL: Tai Chi and fall reductions in older adults: A randomized controlled trial. J Gerontol Ser A Biol Sci Med Sci 2005;60A:187–194.

William W.N. Tsang, PhD, Assistant Professor
Department of Rehabilitation Sciences, The Hong Kong Polytechnic University
Hung Hom, Kowloon, Hong Kong, SAR (China)
Tel. +852 2766 6717, Fax +852 2330 8656, E-Mail rswtsang@polyu.edu.hk

Hong Y (ed): Tai Chi Chuan. State of the Art in International Research.
Med Sport Sci. Basel, Karger, 2008, vol 52, pp 115–123

....

Tai Chi and Balance Control

Alice M.K. Wong[a], *Ching Lan*[b]

[a]Department of Physical Medicine and Rehabilitation, Chang-Gung Memorial
Hospital and Department of Physical Therapy, Post-Graduate Institute of
Rehabilitation Science, Chang-Gung University, [b]Department of Physical Medicine
and Rehabilitation, National Taiwan University Hospital and College of Medicine,
National Taiwan University, Taipei, Taiwan, ROC

Abstract

Balance function begins to decline from middle age on, and poor balance function
increases the risk of fall and injury. Suitable exercise training may improve balance function
and prevent accidental falls. The coordination of visual, proprioceptive, vestibular and musculoskeletal system is important to maintain balance. Balance function can be evaluated by
functional balance testing and sensory organization testing. Tai Chi Chuan (TC) is a popular
conditioning exercise in the Chinese community, and recent studies substantiate that TC is
effective in balance function enhancement and falls prevention. In studies utilizing functional balance testing, TC may increase the duration of one-leg standing and the distance of
functional reach. In studies utilizing sensory organization testing, TC improves static and
dynamic balance, especially in more challenging sensory perturbed condition. Therefore, TC
may be prescribed as an alternative exercise program for elderly subjects or balance-impaired
patients. Participants can choose to perform a complete set of TC or selected movements
according to their needs. In conclusion, TC may improve balance function and is appropriate
for implementation in the community.

Copyright © 2008 S. Karger AG, Basel

Balance function is important during sports and daily activities. In elderly
population, poor balance function may result in accidental fall and injuries.
Falls are a major cause of morbidity, hospitalization, and even mortality among
older people. Approximately 30% of those over 65 years of age sustain a fall,
with about half of them having multiple events. About 10–15% of falls result in
serious injuries and in soft tissue injuries. Serious injuries, such as major fracture and traumatic brain injury, may cause complications and even death. From
1996 to 2000, the incidence of hip fracture in Taiwan was 225/100,000 in men

and 505/100,000 in women in individuals 50 years or older. Most of them (89%) received surgical treatment and the economic burden to the society and family was great. Previous studies reported that exercise training can enhance balance function, and it may reduce the rate of falls and fall-related injuries. In recent years, Tai Chi (TC) has acquired attention owning to its potential benefits to physical fitness traits such as aerobic function, muscular strength and flexibility. Recent research also proved the effect of TC in balance promotion and falls prevention. In this chapter, we review the existing literature and introduce the effects of TC on balance function promotion.

Definition and Organization of Balance

Balance is defined as the state of an object when the resultant load acting upon it is zero (Newton's first Law) [1]. Balance is often referred as the ability of maintenance in postural stability of a person not to fall.

In the systematic model, balance is a complex process which depends on the integration of mechanical, sensory, and motor processing strategies to keep stable upright standing. The visual, proprioceptive, and vestibular systems are three sources of afferent information to influence the control of balance which is termed 'sensory organization' [2].

The second component, termed 'muscle coordination', describes the processes which determine the temporal sequencing and the contractile activity in the muscles of legs and trunk to generate the supportive reactions. The motor strategies for perturbation of balance can be initiated by automatic responses by ankle strategy, hip strategy, suspensory strategy or stepping strategy.

The good postural control depends on sensorimotor integration which requires adequate muscle strength, body alignment, flexibility of trunk and limbs, sensory inputs and central processing. Impaired balance and strength of lower extremities were noticed as major risk factors of fall [2].

Evaluation of Balance Function

The popular balance test can be divided into two categories: functional and laboratory-based tests. The functional balance tests are evaluated by one-leg standing test, Tandem stance, Berg balance test, Romberg test, functional reach test, stepping , timed up and go, and lateral stability test. The laboratory-based test is represented by the sensory organization test (SOT), tilt board with sensors and biomechanic analysis with force plate. The SOT was developed by Nashner; the subject's postural control is tested while standing under 6 reduced or conflicting sensory conditions, including combinations of 3 visual conditions (eyes open, eyes closed, sway referenced) with 2 support surface conditions (fixed, sway referenced) and 1 simultaneous perturbation of vision and proprioception condition (eye open with sway vision and sway surface).

TC Exercise and Balance

TC is a traditional Chinese conditioning exercise. The basic forms of TC exercise are a series of graceful movements linked together in a continuous sequence. TC puts emphasis on maintaining a vertical posture with extended head and trunk position, constantly shifting weight from one leg to the other, with a lower center of gravity (knee and hips held in flexion). Shifting of body weight, rotations, and standing on a single leg with push-pull movements of upper extremities are repeatedly practiced while performing TC. Thus, delicate joint control and muscle coordination are facilitated to achieve good balance control of the body.

Studies of TC and Balance Control

Functional Balance Testing
TC is an exercise with slow motion, and hence the duration of one-leg standing is significantly prolonged. Tse and Bailey [3] were the first to evaluate the beneficial effects of TC on balance. One-leg standing with eyes open and closed was tested in 18 elderly subjects (9 TC practitioners and 9 nonpractitioners), and the TC group practiced this exercise for at least 1 year. The TC group displayed significantly longer one-leg standing duration than the control group in both legs.

TC is practiced at very slow speed, thus biomechanically TC gait may be different from normal walking. In a recent study, Mao et al. [4] compared the duration of one-leg standing during TC practice with that of one-leg standing during normal walking. The duration of each one-leg stance was longer during TC than during walking (1.95 vs. 0.4 s). Additionally, the medial-lateral and anteroposterior displacements of the center of pressure (COP) were increased during TC practice. Balancing on one leg for longer periods required more muscle activities [5], thus TC gait may help managing the activities encountered in daily activities, and may reduce the risk of falls in the elderly.

TC is also effective in improving functional balance in patients with arthritis. Song et al. [6] randomized 72 older women with arthritis into a TC group and a control group. After 12 weeks of training, the TC group displayed significant improvement in dynamic balance measured by one-leg standing test. Further, the arthritic symptom and physical function were also improved.

Most studies found a 12-week TC program is sufficient to improve balance function. In a recent study, however, Zhang et al. [7] reported that an 8-week simplified TC program (1 h daily) was effective in enhancing dynamic balance, flexibility and reduce fear of falls. Tsang and Hui-Chan [8] compared the effect of a 4-week and an 8-week TC training on balance control in elderly individuals. After 4 or 8 weeks of TC training, participants showed similar improvements in vestibular ratio and directional control in the limits of stability test. Further, the improved balance from week 4 was comparable to that of experienced TC practitioners. The results implied that even a 4-week intensive TC program was sufficient to improve balance function in elderly subjects.

Most studies applied TC in elderly population, but TC is also effective to enhance balance in middle-aged individuals. Jacobson et al. [9] reported that TC could improve balance, kinesthetic sense, and strength in younger populations. Thornton et al. [10] also reported a 12-week Yang TC program (3 times per week) could significantly improve functional reach in women aged 35–55 years.

Sensory Organization Testing

Wolf et al. [11] reported the effect of TC training in an Atlanta subgroup of the clinical trial of FICSIT (Fraility and Injuries: Cooperative Studies of Intervention Techniques). Seventy-two inactive older adults over the age of 70 were randomly assigned to three groups, TC, balance training and educational group. The TC group practices 10 forms of Yang's style twice weekly for 15 weeks, while the balance training group received computerized balance training. Testing analyzed postural sway under four conditions: standing with eyes open, standing with eyes closed, toes up with eyes open, toes up with eyes closed. The results showed that the balance training group had significant improvement in postural stability, but the TC group and the control groups did not. However, the TC group displayed less fear of falling and experienced a delayed onset of falls.

Wolfson's group reported the result of a Connecticut subgroup in the FICSIT study. One hundred and ten healthy elderly with a mean age of 80 years participated in a 3-month balance training and then received 6 months of TC training. Computerized and nonplatform balance training significantly improved all balance measures (loss of balance, single stance time, voluntary limits of stability, isokinetic torque of lower extremities and gait velocity), and subsequent TC training could maintain the gains from balance training.

Studies of postural control and balance in TC have flourished in the recent decade. Some studies reported TC had a significant effect on strength enhancement of lower extremities for improvement of postural stability [9, 12]. Many studies using the SOT proved the effectiveness of TC on static and dynamic balance [9, 13]. Moreover, several randomized control studies also reported the beneficial effects of TC on balance control in at-risk or ill elderly individuals [14, 15]. The results can be summarized according to different sensory systems.

Balance and the Proprioceptive System

Wong et al. [13] utilized the SOT to evaluate 25 elderly long-term TC practitioners and 14 controls. In static postural balance testing, there was no difference between the TC and the control group in simple conditions. In more challenging conditions, the TC group showed better postural control in the condition with simultaneous perturbation of vision and proprioception (i.e. eyes open with sway surface, sway vision with sway surface). Further, the TC group also performed better in rhythmic forward-backward weight shifting test.

Tsang and Hui-chan [16] examined the knee proprioception in 42 elderly subjects by using the passive knee joint reposition test. The results displayed that TC practitioners had better knee joint proprioceptive acuity than control subjects. Because TC puts a great emphasis on exact joint positions and directions, the practice of TC may improve the sense of position in lower extremities. In another study, Tsang and Hui-Chan [8] reported that TC practitioners had similar knee joint proprioceptive acuity. Similarly, Xu et al. [5] measured ankle and knee joint kinesthesis by detecting the threshold of passive movement in elderly TC practitioners, swimmers/runners, and controls. TC practitioners not only showed better proprioception at the ankle and knee joints than the controls, but also showed better ankle kinesthesis than swimmers/runners.

In a recent study, Fong and Ng [17] compared long-term (practice for 1–3 years) and short-term (practice for 3 months) TC training for middle-aged and older individuals. The long-term TC training group exhibited significantly faster reflex reaction time in hamstrings and gastrocnemius and a longer balance time on a tilt board than the short-term TC training and the control groups. Both the long-term and short-term training groups had significantly better knee joint position accuracy than the control group. The results implied that both long-term and short-term TC training might improve joint position sense, but only long-term TC training could significantly enhance dynamic standing balance.

In a recent study, Woo et al. [18] randomized 90 men and 90 women into 3 groups (TC, resistance training and control). The TC group practiced simplified 24-form TC three times per week for 12 months; while the resistance training group underwent Thera-Band exercise with medium strength. However, no significant changes in balance, muscle strength and flexibility were observed in men and women for either exercise group compared with controls.

Balance and the Visual System

Lin and Wong [19] used the SOT to evaluate 14 elderly TC practitioners and 14 healthy elderly subjects. The results showed that they had better postural stability at sway-referenced vision and fixed support, and even at the more challenging condition of sway-referenced vision and support than the control group. Tsang et al. [20] investigated elderly TC practitioners using the SOT and found that their visual ratio was higher than that of nonpractitioners, and even comparable to the ratio of the young subjects. The results implied long-term practice of TC improved balance control in the elderly population and there was an increased reliance on the visual system during stance. In addition, elderly TC practitioners attained the same level of balance control as young subjects when standing in reduced or conflicting sensory conditions.

Balance and the Vestibular System

Wong et al. [13] found that elderly TC practitioners had better maximal stability and average velocity than the controls under the condition of sway-referenced support and eyes closed (ECSS). Long-term TC practitioners (practiced TC for 20.4 ± 7 years) used more ankle strategy under the condition of ECSS than the short-term TC practitioners (practiced TC for less than 3 years). Tsang and Hui-Chan [21] proposed that practicing TC involved head movements that stimulate the vestibular system. By using the SOT, the elderly TC practitioners attained a higher vestibular ratio than the controls under the condition of ECSS.

TC may be applied to patients with balance disorders. Hain et al. [22] reported the effect of TC on 22 patients with balance disorders. Patients learned 8 TC movements and practiced at home everyday at least for 30 min. After 2 months, significant improvements were found in the SOT and the Dizziness Handicap Inventory scores. McGibbon et al. [14] also reported a randomized clinical trial in older adults with vestibulopathy. Thirty-six subjects were randomized into a 10-week program of vestibular rehabilitation or TC exercise. The improvements of the TC group were associated with reorganized neuromuscular pattern in lower extremities, while the vestibular rehabilitation group only had better control of upper body motion to minimize loss of balance.

Tsang and Hui-Chan [23] compared the effects of vestibular stimulation on standing balance between older TC practitioners and sedentary controls. Subjects sat on a chair with their heads fixed at $30°$ of flexion, and experienced clockwise whole body rotation at $80°$/s for 60 s with eyes closed. After rotation, subjects stood on a forced platform with eyes closed, and maintained their static balance. The TC group showed significantly smaller increases in total sway path, peak amplitude, and mean velocity of body sway in the anterioposterior direction than the control group.

Balance and Muscle Strength or Flexibility

TC is performed in a semi-squat posture with head and body rotations, and changes the base of support from double stance to single-leg standing. Various degrees of concentric and eccentric contractions of leg muscles are performed during the practice. Therefore, TC could significantly enhance muscular strength and endurance in the lower extremities. Lan et al. [12] evaluated the effect of a 6-month TC program in older individuals. In the male group, the concentric peak torque of knee extensor increased by 15.1–20.0%, while the eccentric peak torque increased by 15.1–23.7%. In the male TCC group, the endurance ratio of knee extensor also increased by 10.3–13.5%. In the female group, the concentric peak torque of knee extensor increased by 13.5–24.2%, while the eccentric peak torque increased by 18.3–23.8%. The female TCC group also showed a 10.1–14.6% increase in the endurance ratio of knee extensor. Lan et al. [12] reported that a 12-month TC program could significantly improve muscle strength of knee extensors/flexors and thoracolumbar flexibility. Other studies also mentioned that TC increases flexibility of the knee [24] and trunk [7].

Biomechanical Benefits of TC

Wu and Hitt [25] measured the ground reaction force, COP and plantar pressure patterns under the stance foot of TC. The results showed TC gait had a low impact force, a fairly evenly distributed body weight between the forefoot and rearfoot regions, and a large medial-lateral displacement of the foot COP. The low-impact force may be attributed to the slow speed of TC and the coordinated activities of the muscles of lower extremities. In addition, maintaining foot COP in the mid-foot region and keeping the plantar pressure equally distributed between the forefoot and rearfoot require a precise control of the neuromuscular system, and the biomechanical characteristics of TC may be helpful to functional balance.

Most studies investigated the effect of TC on balance function, but few studies examined the effect of TC on biomechanical responses to large, fast walking perturbation in balance-impaired seniors. Because the inability to recover from a slip or trip during walking accounts for the majority of falls, to examine the training effect on recovery during a slip while walking may be better than balance testing in standing position.

Conclusion

TC exercise is effective in the organization of proprioceptive, visual and vestibular systems, which are important to maintain balance and prevent falls. Additionally, TC is practiced at very slow speed with a semi-squat posture, thus it improves muscle strength of the lower extremities. TC gait has a low-impact force, and the body weight is evenly distributed on the forefoot and rearfoot regions. In this unique posture, delicate neuromuscular coordination is needed. TC can be applied not only to healthy middle-aged or elderly individuals, but also to frail or balance-impaired seniors. A 4-week short-term but intensive program appears to be sufficient to improve the balance function. Although most TC studies reported beneficial effects on balance function, the training protocol, i.e. style, duration, number of movements, was variable among these studies. In future studies, a simple and standardized TC program may be needed to facilitate learning in the community.

References

1   Baloh RW, Corona S, Jacobson KM, Enrietto JA, Bell T: A prospective study of posturography in normal older people. J Am Geriatr Soc 1998;46:438–443.
2   Nashner LM: Evaluation of postural stability, movement and control; in Hasson SM (ed): Clinical exercise physiology. St. Louis, Mosby, 1994, pp 199–234.
3   Tse SK, Bailey DM: T'ai chi and postural control in the well elderly. Am J Occup Ther 1992;46:295–300.
4   Mao DW, Li JX, Hong Y: The duration and plantar pressure distribution during one-leg stance in Tai Chi exercise. Clin Biomech 2006;21:640–645.
5   Xu D, Hong Y, Li J, Chank: Effect of Tai Chi exercise on proprioception of ankle and knee joint in old people. Br J Sport Med 2004;38:50–54.
6   Song R, Lee EO, Lam P, Bae SC: Effects of Tai Chi exercise on pain, balance, muscle strength, and perceived difficulties in physical functioning in older women with osteoarthritis. J Rheumatol 2003;30:2039–2044.
7   Zhang JG, Ishikawa-Takata K, Yamazaki H, Morita T, Ohta T: The effect of Tai Chi Chuan on physiological function and fear of falling in the less robust elderly: an intervention study for preventing falls. Arch Gerontol Geriatr 2006;42:107–116.
8   Tsang WW, Hui-Chan CW: Effect of 4- and 8-wk intensive Tai Chi training on balance control in the elderly. Med Sci Sports Exerc 2004;36:648–657.
9   Jacobson BH, Chen HC, Cashel C: The effect of Tai Chi Chuan training on balance, kinesthetic sense, and strength. Percept Mot Skills 1997;84:27–33.
10 Thornton EW, Skyes KS, Tang WK: Health benefits of Tai Chi exercise: improved balance and blood pressure in middle-aged women. Health Promot Intern 2004;19:33–38.
11 Wolf SL, Barnhart HX, Ellison GL, Coogler CE: The effect of Tai Chi Quan and computerized balance training on postural stability in older subjects. Atlanta FICSIT Group. Frailty and Injuries:Cooperative Studies on Intervention Techniques. Phys Ther 1997;77:371–381.

12   Lan C, Lai JS, Chen SY, et al: 12-month Tai Chi training in the elderly: its effect on health fitness. Med Sci Sports Exerc 1998;30:345–351.
13   Wong AM, Lin YC, Chou SW, Tang FT, Wong PY: Coordination exercise and postural stability in elderly people: effect of Tai Chi Chuan. Arch Phys Med Rehabil 2001;82:608–612.
14   McGibbon CA, Krebs DE, Parker SW, Scarborough DM, Wayne PM, Wolf SL: Tai Chi and vestibular rehabilitation improve vestibulopathic gait via different neuromuscular mechanisms: preliminary report. BMC Neurol 2005;5:3.
15   Faber MJ, Bosscher RJ, Chin A, Paw MJ, van Wieringen PC: Effects of exercise programs on falls and mobility in frail and pre-frail older adults: a multicenter randomized controlled trial. Arch Phys Med Rehabil 2006;87:885–896.
16   Tsang WW, Hui-Chan CW: Effects of Tai Chi on joint proprioception and stability limits in elderly subjects. Med Sci Sports Exerc 2003;35:1962–1971.
17   Fong SM, Ng GY: The effects on sensorimotor performance and balance with Tai Chi training. Arch Phys Med Rehabil 2006;87:82–87.
18   Woo J, Hong A, Lau E, Lynn H: A randomized controlled trial of Tai Chi and resistance exercise on bone health, muscle strength and balance in community-living elderly people. Age Aging 2007;36:262–268.
19   Lin YC, Wong AMK, Chou SW, Tang FT, Wong PY: The effect of Tai Chi Chuan on Postural Stability in the elderly: Preliminary Report. Chang Gung Med J 2000;23:197–204.
20   Tsang WW, Wong VS, Fu SN, Hui-Chan CW: Tai Chi improves standing balance control under reduced or conflicting sensory conditions. Arch Phys Med Rehabil 2004;85:129–137.
21   Tsang WW, Hui-Chan CW: Standing balance after vestibular stimulation in Tai Chi-practicing and nonpracticing healthy older adults. Arch Phys Med Rehabil 2006;87:546–553.
22   Hain TC, Fuller L, Weil L, Kotsias J: Effects of Tai Chi on balance. Arch Otolaryngol Head Neck Surg 1999;125:1191–1195.
23   Tsang WW, Hui-Chan CW: Standing balance after vestibular stimulation in Tai Chi practicing and nonpracticing healthy older adults. Arch Phys Med Rehabil 2006;87:546–553.
24   Taylor-Piliae RE, Haskell WL, Stotts NA, Froelicher ES: Improvement in balance, strength, and flexibility after 12 weeks of Tai chi exercise in ethnic Chinese adults with cardiovascular disease risk factors. Altern Ther Health Med 2006;12:50–58.
25   Wu G, Hitt J: Ground contact characteristics of Tai Chi gait. Gait Posture 2005;22:32–39.

Alice M.K. Wong, MD
Professor and Chair of Postgraduate
Department of Physical Medicine and Rehabilitation, Chang-Gung Memorial Hospital
199 Tun-Hwa N Rd
Taipei 105, Taiwan (ROC)
Tel. +886 3 211 8800, ext. 5439, Fax +886 3 211 8700, E-Mail walice@adm.cgmh.org.tw

Hong Y (ed): Tai Chi Chuan. State of the Art in International Research.
Med Sport Sci. Basel, Karger, 2008, vol 52, pp 124–134

....

Tai Chi and Falls Prevention in Older People

Peter A. Harmer[a], Fuzhong Li[b]

[a]Excercise Science, Sports Medicine, Willamette University, Salem, Oreg., and
[b]Oregon Research Institute, Eugene, Oreg., USA

Abstract

Background: Considerable research evidence has been accumulated since 1990 that practicing Tai Chi can ameliorate multiple characteristics in older adults that place them at increased risk of falling, including poor balance, loss of strength, limited flexibility, and fear of falling. However, relatively few studies have directly examined the influence of Tai Chi practice on falls in this population. **Results:** Nine randomized controlled trials utilizing Tai Chi (n = 6), or Tai Chi-inspired exercise (n = 3), were published between 1996 and July, 2007. The studies varied considerably on study settings, participant characteristics, sample size, type of Tai Chi intervention, length of intervention and quality of the study design. Of the six studies that used Tai Chi forms, three showed significant improvement in fall-related outcomes. One study using Tai Chi-inspired exercise also had a significant fall-related outcome. **Conclusion:** Despite the evidence demonstrating the beneficial influence of Tai Chi practice on known risk factors for falling in older adults, evidence indicating an actual impact on falls-related outcomes is equivocal. More large-scale, longitudinal studies with consistent intervention parameters and clinically meaningful outcome variables are needed to a clarify the role of Tai Chi in effective falls prevention programs. The recent development of a standardized, research-to-practice Tai Chi falls prevention program may be an important step in this process.

The well-documented fiscal and quality-of-life costs to individuals, healthcare systems and society related to premature morbidity and mortality from falling in older adults are likely to continue to rise as a result of the worldwide growth in the proportion of the population aged over 65 as well as their increasing longevity. Given these conditions, identifying efficacious, cost-effective interventions to reduce the risk of falling, the number of falls, or the number of injurious falls, in this population is imperative. Although falling in older adults is a multifactorial phenomenon [1], involving both internal (i.e. physiological/psychological deficits) and external (e.g. uneven/slippery surfaces, poor lighting) factors [2], the identification of impaired gait, poor balance, and muscle weakness as significant risk factors highlights the importance of exercise programs aimed at ameliorating these characteristics. Essential features of Tai Chi, including its slow, low-impact movements, requiring multidirectional weight shifting, single and double leg weight-bearing, and awareness of alignment, clearly challenge these functional limitations in older adults in a controlled and progressive fashion, as shown in multiple studies [see the chapters by Lan et al., pp. 12–19; Xu et al., pp. 20–29; Wu, pp. 30–39; Taylor-Piliae, pp. 40–53; Thornton, pp. 54–63; Li et al., pp. 77–86; Gatts, pp. 87–103; Tsang and Hui-Chan, pp. 104–114; Wong and Lan, pp. 115–123].

Although a logical extension of the findings of improved balance and strength in older adults who participated in Tai Chi would be a decrease in the falls-related measures mentioned previously, without well-designed, randomized, controlled trials with falls-related outcomes, it would be difficult to present Tai Chi as an effective falls prevention intervention.

Tai Chi and Fall Prevention

Beginning with the pioneering study by Wolf et al. in 1996 [3], only nine Tai Chi-related randomized controlled trials with fall-related outcomes have appeared in the literature [2–10]. Six of these have used some form of 'pure' Tai Chi as an intervention [3, 5–7, 9, 10]; the remaining studies have involved Tai Chi-'inspired' exercise or a mixed intervention [2, 4, 8]. Despite the theoretical and research support that indicates Tai Chi as a viable mechanism for improving fall-related outcomes in older adults, the results to date have been equivocal. The lack of consistent findings may be due to the large variations in study settings, participant characteristics, sample size, type of Tai Chi intervention, length of intervention and quality of the study design. A summary of study characteristics of the nine papers, in chronological order, is presented in table 1.

To get a clearer picture of the impact of Tai Chi training on fall-related outcomes, it seems useful to divide these trials into groups based on shared characteristics such as the setting or subject inclusion/exclusion criteria. Thus, the nine papers can be categorized into studies of: (a) healthy, community-dwelling older adults with standardized Tai Chi intervention in the research setting [3, 6], (b) healthy, community-dwelling older adults with nonstandardized Tai Chi intervention conducted in community settings [9, 10], (c) older adults specifically at risk for falling based on objective attributes such recent fall episodes,

Table 1. Summary of Tai Chi trials and falls prevention.

Author	Ages	Location	Sample characteristics	Intervention	Frequency	Duration	Falls outcomes
Wolf et al. [3]	≥70 years (mean = 76.2)	USA	Community-living; n = 200 (male = 38; female = 162)	10-form Yang style (n = 72); computerized balance training (n = 64); education control (n = 64)	Tai Chi – 2/week (45 min total); computerized balance training and education control – 1/week	15 weeks	Risk of falls reduced by 47.5% in Tai Chi group (RR = 0.525; 95% CI: 0.321–0.86)
Nowalk et al. [2]	≥65 years (mean = 84)	USA	long-term care facilities; n = 110 (male = 15; female = 95)	Tai Chi/cognitive behavioral/educational program (n = 38); strength and conditioning/educational program (n = 37); educational program control (n = 35)	Tai Chi – 3/week (session length not indicated); strength 3/week (session length not indicated); educational control (frequency and session length not indicated)	52–112 weeks	No significant differences in rate of falls or time to first fall between intervention or control groups
Barnett et al. [4]	≥65 years (mean = 74.9)	Australia	Community-living; n = 163 (male = 54; female = 109)	Multifaceted exercise, incorporating modified Tai Chi (n = 83); control (n = 80)	1 h/week	37 weeks	Rate of falls reduced by 40% in intervention group (IRR = 0.605; 95% CI: 0.36–0.99); lower proportion for ≥2 falls (RR = 0.44; 95% CI: 0.21–0.96)

Study	Age	Country	Setting	Intervention	Protocol	Duration	Outcomes
Wolf et al. [5]	≥70 years (mean = 80.9)	USA	Nursing home residents; n = 311 (male = 20; female = 291)	Specifically selected 6-form Tai Chi (n = 145); wellness education (n = 141)	Tai Chi – 2/week (progressing from 60 min to 90 min over the study); wellness education – 1 h/week	48 weeks	No significant differences in rate of falls between groups; for participants with previous fall fractures, TC group had significantly lower fall risk (RR = 0.58; 95% CI: 0.38–0.9)
Li et al. [6]	≥70 years (mean = 77.5)	USA	Community-living; n = 256 (male = 77; female = 179)	24-form Yang-style (n = 125); stretching control (n = 131)	Both groups – 1-hour classes; 3/week	26 weeks	Significantly fewer falls in TC group (p = 0.007); significantly lower risk for moderate (RR = 0.31; 95% CI: 0.12–0.84) and severe (RR = 0.28; 95% CI: 0.09–0.86) injurious falls in TC group
Choi et al. [7]	≥60 years (mean = 77.8)	Korea	Residential care facility; n = 68 (male = 15; female = 44)	12-form Sun style (n = 29); control (n = 30)	35-min classes; 3/week	12 weeks	No significant differences in fall episodes
Faber et al. [8]	≥63 years (mean = 84.9)	Netherlands	Nursing home residents; n = 238 (male = 50; female = 188)	Tai Chi-inspired exercises (n = 80); functional walking (n = 66); control (n = 92)	90 min/session (30 min socializing component); 1/week for 4 weeks; 2/week for 16 weeks	20 weeks	No significant differences in percentage of participants who fell or time to first fall.

Table 1. (continued)

Author	Ages	Location	Sample characteristics	Intervention	Frequency	Duration	Falls outcomes
Lin et al. [9]	≥65 years	Taiwan	Community-living; n = 1,288 (male = 737; female = 551)	13-form Chen style (n = 88); education program (n = 1,288)	1 h/class; 6/week	52 weeks	No significant differences in occurrence of injurious falls
Voukelatos et al. [10]	≥60 years (mean = 69)	Australia	Community-living; n = 702 (male = 115; female = 587)	Community-based classes – various Tai Chi styles (83% Sun style; 3% Yang style; 14% mixture of Tai Chi styles; n = 353); wait-list control (n = 349)	1 h/week	16 weeks	Hazard ratio for 2 or more falls in TC group significantly different compared to control (HR = 0.33; 95% CI: 0.14–0.78) at 16 weeks. At 8 weeks postintervention follow-up, significantly lower risk for multiple falls in TC group (RR = 0.54; 95% CI: 0.28–0.96); and significantly lower fall rate (IRR = 0.67; 95% CI: 0.46–0.96)

impaired balance or hypotension [4, 5, 7], and (d) residents of long-term care facilities [2, 5, 7, 8].

Healthy, Community-Dwelling Adults in Research Settings

Well-controlled studies with strong internal validity are important in establishing the viability of causal relationships in studies of human function. Significant findings provide justification for expanding research parameters, such as participant characteristics and intervention attributes, to gain a more complete understanding of the scope of the relationship.

Wolf et al. [3] compared the efficacy of two methods of exercise on falls. Community-living healthy adults (n = 200) were randomized to Tai Chi training, computerized balance training or an educational control group. The Tai Chi intervention was a simplified 10-form program that met two times per week for 45 min of total individualized contact time. Participants in the computerized balance training group had one 45 min session per week. Results of this 15-week trial showed that Tai Chi participants experienced a significant reduction (by about 47%) in the rate of falls compared to the exercise control participants in follow-up that ranged from 7 to 20 months.

Li et al. [6] confirmed the general findings of Wolf and his colleagues. Participants (n = 256) were randomly assigned to a Tai Chi or stretching control group. The Tai Chi intervention used the 24-form Yang style, with 1-hour classes meeting three times per week for 24 weeks. The stretching control met for the same time. At the end of a 6-month intervention, significantly fewer falls (38 vs. 73), and lower proportions of fallers (28 vs. 46%), and injurious falls (7 vs. 18%) were observed in the Tai Chi condition, compared to a low-impact stretching control condition. Overall, the risk of multiple falls in the Tai Chi group was 55% lower than that of the stretching controls. Of equal importance, intervention gains in these measures were maintained at a 6-month postintervention follow-up in the Tai Chi group.

Healthy, Community-Dwelling Adults in Community Settings

Laboratory-based randomized, controlled trials are conducted with rigorous predefined study conditions, which limit the applicability of the findings to nonequivalent settings. Community-based studies are necessary to clarify the generalizability, or robustness, of the causal relationship under investigation.

A study by Lin et al. [9] involved six villages from the same province in Taiwan. Two of the villages were selected to support a 1-hour per day, 6 day per week Tai Chi class conducted in public spaces while the remaining villages were used as controls. However, all villages received 1 year of public falls prevention education prior to the Tai Chi intervention. Moreover, 5 persons from control villages practiced Tai Chi and were included in analyses of Tai Chi practitioners (n = 88). In the final analyses comparing the Tai Chi practitioners, inhabitants of the villages in which the Tai Chi program was offered, and the control villagers, no significant differences were found in the rate of injurious falls.

Voukelatos et al. [10] assigned 702 community-dwelling adults aged 60 and older to participate in a 1-hour class, 1 day a week for 16 weeks or to a 24 weeks wait-list control group. Existing community-based Tai Chi classes were utilized and represented a variety of styles. No modifications were imposed by the investigators but participants were required to pay a modest fee as an incentive to enhance attendance. Fall data were evaluated at the end of the 16-week program and at an 8-week postintervention follow-up. Although the incident rate ratio was not significant at the end of the intervention, it was significant at the 8-week follow-up, with the Tai Chi group demonstrating a 33% lower rate of falling than the control group. However, the hazard ratio for 2 or more falls was significantly different between the Tai Chi and control groups at both 16 and 24 weeks (HR = 0.33 at both time points).

Older Adults Specifically at Risk for Falling

Although age is a known risk factor for falling, not all older adults are at the same risk. Several researchers have attempted to determine the utility of Tai Chi in reducing the risk of falling in the most vulnerable of older adults by specifically targeting those at highest risk, that is, those with multiple specific high-risk characteristics, including a history of recent falls, impaired balance, lower limb weakness or gait disturbances.

In a community-based program in Australia, Barnett et al. [4] randomly assigned 163 high-risk patients referred from physiotherapy clinics to either a 1 h per week structured exercise class for 1 year or a falls prevention education control group. The exercise intervention consisted of in-class and at-home activities designed to improve strength, aerobic capacity, coordination and balance. Modified Tai Chi exercises were used as part of the program aimed at coordination and balance improvement. The exercise group also received the falls prevention educational material. The exercise group had a significantly lower fall rate than the control (IRR = 0.605; 95% CI = 0.36–0.99) as well as a significantly lower proportion of participants who experienced 2 or more falls (RR = 0.44; 95% CI = 0.21–0.96). There was no significant difference between groups on the rate of injurious falls.

Wolf et al. [5] extended their previous work on Tai Chi and falling in older adults by recruiting older adults who were less robust (that is, transitioning to frailty). Residents from 20 nursing homes (n = 311) were randomized into an 'intense' Tai Chi group or a wellness education control. The Tai Chi group met two times per week for 48 weeks, and practiced a simplified 6-form Tai Chi, increasing the training load from 1 h per class initially to 90 min per class at the end of the study. The wellness education control met for 1 h per week. Although there was no significant difference between groups on the risk of falling over the course of the study, fall data from month 4 through month 12 showed a significantly reduced risk of falls in the Tai Chi group compared with the control group (RR = 0.54; 95% CI = 0.36–0.81). Moreover, there was a significantly lower fall rate for Tai Chi participants without a previous fall fracture compared to those in the control group (RR = 0.58; 95% CI = 0.38–0.90).

Most recently, Choi [7] led a study of at-risk nursing home residents (n = 68) in Korea, who were randomly assigned to a standardized 12-form Sun style Tai Chi class or a control group. The Tai Chi class met for 35 min, three times per week for 12 weeks. No significant differences were found between groups for fall episodes.

Residents of Long-Term Care Facilities

Being a resident of a nursing home or long-term care facility is a significant risk factor for falling, with the rate of falling in nursing home residents approximately double that of community-dwelling older adults. These settings also produce more serious injurious falls [11, 12]. However, few studies have looked at Tai Chi interventions in this high-risk population. In addition to the studies of Wolf et al. [5] and Choi et al. [7], discussed in the previous section, which involved high-risk nursing home residents, only two studies of healthy nursing home residents (i.e. those without specified additional risk factors for falling) have been conducted.

Nowalk et al. [2] recruited 110 residents from two senior housing facilities to participate in FallsFREE, a study of three falls prevention interventions: (a) educational programs, including walking and medication management (this group served as the control), (b) educational programs plus 'individualized, progressive strength training and conditioning', and (c) educational programs, behavioral-cognitive training, and Tai Chi (conducted three times per week. However, neither the length of each class nor the type of Tai Chi is specified). No significant differences were found between groups on either rate of falls or time to first fall.

Faber et al. [8] restricted exclusion criteria for participants in their study of two falls prevention interventions in the Netherlands to 'enable the generalizability of the results'. Residents of long-term care centers (n = 238) were assigned to: (a) control group, (b) a Functional Walking group, with a focus on balance and functional strength, or (c) an In Balance program, initially incorporating therapeutic elements of Tai Chi, progressing to a simplified form of Tai Chi, among other exercises. The workloads for both interventions were progressively increased from one, 90-min session per week for 4 weeks, to two, 90-min sessions per week for 16 weeks. However, 30 min of each session was devoted to socialization. No significant differences were found for the fall incidence rate between groups.

Summary of Findings

Despite the differences in methodology, conditions and results in the randomized controlled trials examining the influence of Tai Chi on fall-related outcomes, several overarching conclusions seem warranted: (a) Tai Chi is an efficacious falls prevention intervention in health, community-dwelling older adults [3, 6, 10], (b) currently there is little evidence that Tai Chi is efficacious in falls prevention in specific high-risk populations [2, 4, 5, 7, 8], (c) programs based on standard Tai Chi forms are more likely to be effective than those utilizing Tai Chi 'inspired' exercises [2, 3, 6, 8, 10], and (d) a coordinated, systematic research agenda is required if the conditions under which, and the populations for whom, Tai Chi can be advocated to reliably improve fall-related outcomes are to be identified.

Translating Research to Practice

Although the findings of the Tai Chi trials are mixed, there is sufficient evidence to indicate that Tai Chi can improve fall-related outcomes in older adults. However, as Close [13] argues, the 'real challenge is ... to ensure that clinical trial data can be successfully translated and applied to the populations who stand to benefit the most from the intervention'. To date, only Li et al. [6] have attempted to fill this research-to-practice gap. Drawing on the essential elements of their successful intervention, they utilized a two-stage process to: (a) develop 'a program package that is content appropriate, attractive to potential clients, and logistically practical' [14], and (b) implement and evaluate the resulting program in the field [15]. The first objective was achieved through a mixed qualitative and quantitative process involving input from experts in public health, epidemiology, physical and occupational therapy, Tai Chi instruction, service evaluation and senior services provision. The utility of the resulting program, Tai Chi – Moving for Better Balance, was evaluated through the RE-AIM framework [16, 17] in six senior centers in Oregon, USA. Findings indicate the program to be logistical feasible, with high client satisfaction, significant impact on participant characteristics such as balance, and promising results for falls attenuation. The program has been adopted by a state agency and disseminated to senior service providers throughout the state.

Conclusions

There is no doubt that Tai Chi is effective in enhancing a wide range of physiological and psychological characteristics in older adults, including some, such as impaired balance and poor lower extremity strength, which have been identified as risk factors for falling. However, the research evidence on the efficacy of Tai Chi practice on fall-related outcomes is problematic. Currently, there are still too few randomized controlled trials, which are too fragmented, to gain a complete picture of the relationship between Tai Chi and falls prevention. To date, only Wolf et al. [3, 5] has attempted anything like an extension study, and only Li [6, 14, 15] has developed a research-to-practice translation of a successful Tai Chi intervention.

The fact that the existing studies have come from four continents indicates the widespread belief in the possibilities of Tai Chi in reducing fall-related risk in older adults and highlights the opportunity for collaborative research to identify the appropriate combination(s) of program features and participant characteristics for best outcomes [18]. Systematic, progressive explorations of features of the Tai Chi-falls relationship such as optimal style, frequency, duration, and intensity parameters for varying populations, and use of consistent, clinically relevant falls-related outcomes [19] are imperative if the full potential of Tai Chi to positively impact fall-related morbidity and mortality in older adults is to be realized.

References

1 Cumming RG: Intervention strategies and risk-factor modification for falls prevention: A review of recent intervention studies. Clin Geriatr Med 2002;18:175–189.
2 Nowalk MP, Prendergast JM, Bayles CM, D'Amico FJ, Colvin GC: A randomized trial of exercise programs among older individuals living in two long-term care facilities: The FallsFREE program. J Am Geriatr Soc 2001;49:859–865.
3 Wolf SL, Barnhart HX, Kutner NG, McNeely E, Coogler C, Xu T; Atlanta FICSIT Group: Reducing frailty and falls in older persons: An investigation of Tai Chi and computerized balance training. J Am Geriatr Soc 1996;44:489–497.
4 Barnett A, Smith B, Lord SR, Williams M, Baumand A: Community-based group exercise improves balance and reduces falls in at-risk older people: A randomized controlled trial. Age Ageing 2003;32:407–414.
5 Wolf SL, Sattin RW, Kutner M, O'Grady M, Greenspan AI, Gregor RJ: Intense Tai Chi exercise training and fall occurrences in older, transitionally frail adults: A randomized, controlled trial. J Am Geriatr Soc 2003;51:1693–1701.
6 Li F, Harmer P, Fisher KJ, McAuley E, Chaumeton N, Eckstrom E, Wilson NL: Tai Chi and fall reductions in older adults: A randomized controlled trial. J Gerontol Med Sci 2005;60A:66–71.
7 Choi JH, Moon J-S, Song R: Effects of Sun-style Tai Chi exercise on physical fitness and fall prevention in fall-prone older adults. J Adv Nurs 2005;51:150–157.
8 Faber MJ, Bosscher RJ, Chin MJ, Paauw A, van Wieringen PC: Effects of exercise program on falls and mobility in frail and pre-frail older adutls: A multicenter randomized controlled trial. Arch Phys Med Rehabil 2006;87:885–896.

9   Lin M-R, Hwang H-F, Wang Y-W, Chang S-H, Wolf SL: Community-based Tai Chi and its effects on injurious falls, balance, gait, and fear of falling in older people. Phys Therapy 2006;86: 1189–1201.

10 Voukelatos A, Cumming RG, Lord SR, Rissel C: A randomized, controlled trial of Tai Chi for the prevention of falls: The Central Sydney Tai Chi trial. J Am Geriatr Soc DOI: 10.1111/j.1532–5415. 2007.01244.x.

11 Rubenstein LZ, Josephson KR, Robbins AS: Falls in the nursing home. Ann Intern Med 1994; 121:442–451.

12 US Centers for Disease Control and Prevention. Falls in nursing homes Fact Sheet. Available at: www.cdc.gov/ncipc/factsheets/nursing.htm. Accessed on June 20, 2007.

13 Close JCT: Prevention of falls – a time to translate evidence into practice. Age Ageing 2005;34: 98–100.

14 Li F, Harmer P, Mack KA, Sleet D, Fisher KJ, Kohn MA, Millet LM, Sutton B, Tompkins Y: Tai Chi – Moving for Better Balance – Development of a community-based falls prevention program. J Phys Act Health 2007, in press.

15 Li F, Harmer P, Mack KA, Sleet D, Fisher KJ, Kohn MA, Millet LM, Sutton B, Tompkins Y: Translation of an effective Tai Chi intervention into a community-based falls prevention program. Am J Public Health 2008, in press.

16 Glasgow RE, Vogt TM, Boles SM: Evaluating the public health impact of health promotion interventions: The RE-AIM framework. Am J Public Health 1999;89:1322–1327.

17 Glasgow RE, Emmons KM: How can we increase translation of research into practice? Types of evidence needed. Ann Rev Public Health 2007;28:413–433.

18 Gardner MM, Robertson MC, Campbell AJ: Exercise in preventing falls and fall related injuries in older people: A review of randomised controlled trials. Br J Sports Med 2000;34:7–17.

19 Wu G: Evaluation of the effectiveness of Tai Chi for improving balance and preventing falls in the older population – A review. J Am Geriatr Soc 2002;50:746–754.

Peter A. Harmer, PhD, MPH, ATC, FACSM
Exercise Science, Sports Medicine
Willamette University
Salem, OR 973901 (USA)
Tel. +1 503 370 6470, Fax +1 503 370 6379, E-Mail pharmer@willamette.edu

Hong Y (ed): Tai Chi Chuan. State of the Art in International Research.
Med Sport Sci. Basel, Karger, 2008, vol 52, pp 135–145

....

Tai Chi Exercise and the Improvement of Mental and Physical Health among College Students

Yong 'Tai' Wang

Division of Physical Therapy, Georgia State University, Atlanta, Ga., USA

Abstract

Background/Aims: Physical exercise has positive effects on the body as well as on the mind. The purpose of this study was to examine the effects of Tai Chi exercise on college students' perceptions of their physical and mental health. A 3-month Tai Chi intervention (1 h, twice/week) was administrated to 30 college students. The SF-36v2 health survey questionnaire was employed to evaluate the mental health dimension (MHD) and physical health dimension (PHD) before and after the intervention by means of a paired t test ($p < 0.05$). PHD including physical functioning, role physical, bodily pain, general health, and MHD including social functioning, role mental/emotion function, vitality, and perceptions of mental health were assessed. **Results:** Physical measures of bodily pain and general health, and mental measures of role mental/emotion function, vitality, and mental health were significantly improved after Tai Chi intervention. When the overall PHD or MHD scores were evaluated, the MHD increased significantly. **Conclusions:** Tai Chi exercise had positive effects on the self-assessed physical and mental health of college students. Scores on the MHD appeared to be particularly sensitive to change. Colleges/universities might consider offering Tai Chi as a component of their ongoing physical activity programs available to students.

Improving and maintaining mental health and physical health are of concern for everyone. Mental health may be described as a healthy mind with positive attitude and emotional well-being, and with the competence to live a full and creative life and the flexibility to deal with life's inevitable challenges. Physical health may be described as a healthy body with good physical functions and with the competence to fulfill physical demands and challenges in daily life. To balance the busy schedule, heavy work load and mental stress, and all aspects of life – social, physical, spiritual and emotional, it is critical to keep our physical condition and mental status at the optimal level. Numerous studies [1–6] suggested that physical exercises are beneficial to mental health and physical health. Blumenthal et al. [1] concluded that a 16-week aerobic exercise may reduce depression in older adults. Paluska and Schwenk [2] reported that physical activity may play an important role in the management of depression and anxiety, and in general acute anxiety responds better to exercise than chronic anxiety. Vuori [3] stated that there is sufficient scientific evidence recommending regular lifelong physical activity as part of a healthy lifestyle for everyone in order to enhance musculoskeletal health and functions.

Tai Chi Quan is an ancient Chinese martial art and an exercise which is well known for its effects and benefits on balance and coordination training for older populations [4]. Ryan [7] described Tai Chi (Quan) as an exercise, a dance, a method of achieving mental peace and relaxation, and a philosophy of life. Tai Chi may also be thought of as a moving form of yoga and meditation. Compared to some popular exercises, such as walking, jogging, running, or weight lifting, Tai Chi is unique because it is a body-mind exercise, and it has a low impact on the joints. Tai Chi is gaining acceptance in the United States for improving personal health and fitness.

People who practice Tai Chi gain and maintain a healthy body as well as an alert mind, as demonstrated by the ability to concentrate better on routine tasks and to make decisions more effectively [8–11]. However, research on Tai Chi exercise has mainly focused on older adults and the use of Tai Chi for balance and fall prevention [5, 12, 13]. Hain, et al. [6] conducted a study to determine if the practice of Tai Chi significantly improved balance. Twenty-two subjects (16 were 61 years old or older) with mild balance disorders were studied using five measures of balance. The participants underwent 8 weeks of Tai Chi training and practice and the results demonstrated that the posturography test, the Dizziness Handicap Inventory questionnaire, Romberg test and the Medical Outcomes Study Survey scores improved significantly, and findings from this study suggested that Tai Chi practice improved balance for patients with mild balance disorders. Tse and Bailey [12] investigated the potential value of Tai Chi exercise in promoting postural control of the well elderly. The subjects in the study were 65 years of age and older. Comparison of performance on five balance tests between 9 Tai Chi practitioners and nine nonpractitioners demonstrated that the Tai Chi practitioners had significantly better postural control than the sedentary nonpractitioners. Wolf et al. [13] explored the effect of Tai Chi and computerized balance training on postural stability in 24 older adults and concluded that Tai Chi practice may not improve measures of postural stability; however, Tai Chi may gain its success, in part, from promoting confidence without reducing sway rather than primarily facilitating a reduction in sway-based measures.

As observed in the literature, research on Tai Chi exercise has mainly focused on the older population [5, 12, 13]. The effects of Tai Chi exercise on physical and mental health among college students are not well documented. Therefore, the purpose of this study was to determine the effects of Tai Chi, a body-mind harmony exercise, on college students' perceptions of their mental health, and physical health.

Methods

Research Design

A one-group, pre-test, post-test design [14] was utilized in this study. A 3-month series of 1-hour Tai Chi exercise, twice weekly, was the intervention. The multidimensional SF-36v2 health survey questionnaire (refer to appendix) was employed to measure the physical and mental health of the participants before and after the intervention. Paired t test was used to examine the participants' changes of physical and mental health perception before and after Tai Chi practice.

Participants

Thirty college students (11 males and 19 females) attending a large urban university in the southeast volunteered as participants. These college students were enrolled in a university class, 'Tai Chi – A Philosophy for Health and a Therapeutic Exercise,' and the class was offered to graduate and undergraduate students. All participants were informed of the procedures of the experiment and signed a University approved human subject consent form indicating their voluntary participation. All participants were healthy and denied low back dysfunction or any pathological diseases which might negatively impact their performance. The mean age was 24.23 ± 2.74 (standard deviation, SD) years, the mean body height was 170.85 ± 6.12 cm, and the mean body weight was 69.82 ± 18.97 kg. Approximately 70% of these participants were graduate students and 30% were undergraduate students.

Instrumentation

Physical health dimension (PHD) and mental health dimension (MHD) were assessed with the multidimensional SF-36v2 health survey questionnaire [15]. The SF-36v2 contains 36 items and was designed for use in clinical practice, research, health policy evaluations, and general population surveys. The questionnaire covers eight variables of functioning. Physical health measures include:

1   Physical functioning (PF) – limitations in activities such as sports, climbing stairs, walking and dressing;
2   Role physical (RP) – extent to which health interferes with work, housework, or schoolwork;
3   Bodily pain (BP) – extent of BP in the past month;
4   General health (GH) – extent of overall physical distress in the past month.

Mental health measures include:

5   Vitality (VT) – sense of energy and freedom from fatigue;
6   Social functioning (SF) – extent to which health interferes with social activities such as visiting friends or relatives in the past month;

7   Role mental/emotion function (RE) – limitations in usual role activities (work or home) because of emotional problems;
8   General mental health perceptions (MH) – perceptions of mental health.

The SF-36v2 has been used extensively and has good psychometric properties and clinical validity [15]. The scores from these eight variables were generated based on the standardized scoring procedure [16]. The raw scores were transformed to Z scores using the norms (means and SDs) of the US population in 1998 [16]; then, the Z score of each variable was normalized using the following equation: Normalized score $= 50 + Z$ score $\times 10$.

Procedures

An experienced Tai Chi instructor who has taught Tai Chi exercises for many years, including classes at the university level and workshops at national conferences, led this Tai Chi exercise intervention. In the first 2 weeks, the participants learned Tai Chi philosophy, the principles of Tai Chi practice, breathing techniques, and the single Tai Chi forms. In the subsequent 2 weeks, the participants combined the single Tai Chi forms together and completed the psychomotor learning of the Tai Chi 24 forms. For the remainder of the 3 months of the study, the participants practiced the Tai Chi 24 forms with relaxation techniques [17]. Each practice session consisted of 10 min of breathing and stretching exercises followed by 50 min of practice of Tai Chi 24 forms. Participants practiced twice a week on Monday and Wednesday, and make-up sessions were provided on Thursday and Friday for those who missed a regularly scheduled practice session.

Data Analysis

With permission of the Medical Outcomes Trust, a nonprofit organization for the SF-36 Health Survey, the raw data were analyzed using the SF-36 software. The normalized scores of the eight variables and the overall scores in physical and mental dimensions from SF-36v2 were generated and the changes of physical and mental health before and after the Tai Chi intervention were examined by means of paired t test in SPSS [18].

Results

Physical Health Dimension

The results [14] of the comparison of the overall PHD before and after the Tai Chi Quan exercise intervention are presented in figure 1. Of the four physical health variables (PF, RP, BP and GH), two variables, BP and GH were significantly improved ($p < 0.05$) with the Tai Chi intervention. The mean score of BP was improved from 51.41 to 56.60 and the mean of score of GH was improved from 53.20 to 56.45. The overall score of PHD, a combination of the four physical health variables, was enhanced, but did not show statistically significant improvement after the Tai Chi intervention.

Mental Health Dimension

Comparisons of the MHD variables before and after Tai Chi practice are presented in figure 2. Three of the four mental health variables, VT, RE and MH

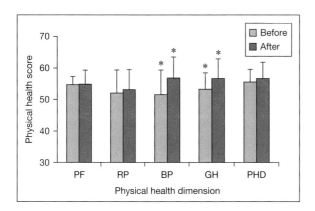

Fig. 1. Comparisons of PHD scores (mean and SD) before and after Tai Chi intervention. *$p < 0.05$, paired t test.

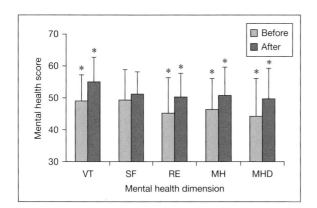

Fig. 2. Comparisons of MHD scores (mean and SD) before and after Tai Chi intervention. *$p < 0.05$, paired t test.

significantly improved ($p < 0.05$) after the Tai Chi intervention. The mean score of VT was improved from 49.06 to 55.00, the mean score of RE was improved from 45.27 to 50.27, and the mean score of MH was improved from 46.26 to 50.76. The overall MHD, a combination of the four mental health variables, showed statistically significant improvement (from 44.26 to 49.71) as well.

Discussion

The results of this study [14] indicated that a Tai Chi program can be beneficial to improving the physical and mental health of college students. In particular, the MHD was particularly sensitive to change in this group, as shown in figure 2. VT, defined as a sense of energy and freedom from fatigue, mental/emotional role function, defined as limitations in usual home or work activities because of emotional problems, and general emotional health all improved as measured at the end of Tai Chi intervention by the SF-36v2. These results initially were surprising to us, given the fact that our sample consisted of healthy graduate and undergraduate students. However, the stresses of daily living, juggling schedules, and making ends meet are factors with which students must constantly grapple. College students, and in particular graduate students, are faced with a myriad of stresses including demands on time, financial issues, peer and academic pressure, and competing role strain. The overall mental health score for the general population in the US is 50 [16]. However, the participants in this study had scores of 44.26 and 49.71 before and after Tai Chi intervention, respectively. These college students had overall mental health scores well below the national average prior to the Tai Chi intervention. The participants' scores closely approximated the national average after the intervention. We think college students, especially graduate students in some intensive academic programs are stressed, and Tai Chi as a mental relaxation exercise has good results of reducing acute stress or anxiety [2] for this group of people. Most participants (approximately 75%) in this Tai Chi program said they felt much more relaxed at the end Tai Chi practice.

The results of the improved mental health scores found in this study are supported by previous studies [2, 10]. Jin [10] examined changes in psychological functioning following participation in Tai Chi exercise and found that participants were less tense, depressed, angry, fatigued and confused. Paluska and Schwenk [2] stated that physical activity may play an important role in the management of mild to moderate mental health anxiety/diseases, and acute anxiety responds better to exercise than chronic anxiety.

In the PHD, in particular the BP variable, defined as the extent of pain in the past month, and the general physical health variable changed significantly, as depicted in figure 1. As with the combined mental health score, the mean physical health score was 50 for the general US population [16]. The participants from this study had scores of 55.47 and 56.70 before and after Tai Chi intervention, well above the mean for the general population. This was to be expected as younger participants have less chronic (physical) disease and are generally in better health.

This study was limited by its nonexperimental design. The lack of a control/comparison group limited its application and a follow-up study comparing Tai Chi with a more traditional exercise program with college students would be

---

helpful. Given the unique mind-body aspects of Tai Chi, it would be particularly interesting to compare the mental health scores between these types of exercise. The majority of students involved in the study was enrolled in the graduate physical therapy program, and as such may be more aware of exercise benefits, and in particular benefits of Tai Chi, or may expect more improvement than students outside of healthcare or physical education programs. A future study would benefit from a more diverse participant pool regarding selected majors and courses of study.

Conclusions

Tai Chi Quan is a unique form of exercise, combining mind and body through a series of low-impact movements. This study offers interesting data for consideration. College students may benefit from regular practice of Tai Chi. Tai Chi may be helpful in mediating emotional and psychological stresses that accompany the life experiences of graduate and undergraduate students. Colleges and universities might consider offering Tai Chi classes as a component of their ongoing physical activity programs available to students.

Appendix

SF-36v2™ Health Survey

This survey asks for your views about your health. This information will help you keep track of how you feel and how well you are able to do your usual activities.

Answer every question by selecting the answer as indicated. If you are unsure about how to answer a question, please give the best answer you can.

---

1) **In general, would you say your health is:**

Excellent	Very good	Good	Fair	Poor
○	○	○	○	○

2) **Compared to one year ago, *how would you rate your health in general now?***

Much better now than one year ago	Somewhat better now than one year ago	About the same as one year ago	Somewhat worse now than one year ago	Much worse now than one year ago
○	○	○	○	○

3) **The following questions are about activities you might do during a typical day.** *Does your health now limit* **you in these activities? If so, how much?** **[Fill in a circle on each line.]**

	Yes, limited a lot	Yes, limited a little	No, not limited at all
a. **Vigorous Activities**, such as running, lifting heavy objects, participating in strenuous sports	O	O	O
b. **Moderate Activities**, such as moving a table, pushing a vacuum cleaner, bowling, or playing golf	O	O	O
c. Lifting or carrying groceries	O	O	O
d. Climbing **several** flights of stairs	O	O	O
e. Climbing **one** flight of stairs	O	O	O
f. Bending, kneeling, or stooping	O	O	O
g. Walking **more than a mile**	O	O	O
h. Walking **several hundred yards**	O	O	O
i. Walking **one hundred yards**	O	O	O
j. Bathing or dressing yourself	O	O	O

4) **During the** *past 4 weeks,* **how much of the time have you had any of the following problems with your work or other regular daily activities** *as a result of your physical health?*

	All of the time	Most of the time	Some of the time	A little of the time	None of the time
a. Cut down on the amount of time you spent on work or other activities	O	O	O	O	O
b. **Accomplished less** than you would like	O	O	O	O	O
c. Were limited in the **kind** of work or other activities	O	O	O	O	O
d. Had **difficulty** performing the work or other activities (for example, it took extra effort)	O	O	O	O	O

5) **During the past 4 weeks, how much of the time have you had any of the following problems with your work or other regular daily activities** *as a result of any emotional problems* **(such as feeling depressed or anxious)?**

	All of the time	Most of the time	Some of the time	A little of the time	None of the time
a. Cut down on the *amount of time* you spent on work or other activities	O	O	O	O	O
b. *Accomplished less* than you would like	O	O	O	O	O

Wang

    c. Did work or activities   ○   ○   ○   ○   ○
        less carefully than usual

6) During the past 4 weeks, to what extent has your physical health or emotional problems interfered with your normal social activities with family, friends, neighbors, or groups?

Not at all	Slightly	Moderately	Quite a bit	Extremely
○	○	○	○	○

7) How much bodily pain have you had during the past 4 weeks?

None	Very Mild	Mild	Moderate	Severe	Very Severe
○	○	○	○	○	○

8) During the past 4 weeks, how much did pain interfere with your normal work (including both work outside the home and housework)?

Not at all	A little bit	Moderately	Quite a bit	Extremely
○	○	○	○	○☆

9) These questions are about how you feel and how things have been with you *during the past 4 weeks*. For each question, please give the one answer that comes closest to the way you have been feeling. How much of the time during the *past 4 weeks*...

	All of the time	Most of the time	Some of the time	A little of the time	None of the time
a. Did you feel full of life?	○	○	○	○	○
b. Have you been very nervous?	○	○	○	○	○
c. Have you felt so down in the dumps that nothing could cheer you up?	○	○	○	○	○
d. Have you felt calm and peaceful?	○	○	○	○	○
e. Did you have a lot of energy?	○	○	○	○	○
f. Have you felt downhearted and depressed?	○	○	○	○	○
g. Did you feel worn out?	○	○	○	○	○
h. Have you been happy?	○	○	○	○	○
i. Did you feel tired?	○	○	○	○	○

10) During the past 4 weeks, how much of the time has your physical health or emotional problems interfered with your social activities (like visiting friends, relatives, etc.)?

All of the time	Most of the time	Some of the time	A little of the time	None of the time
○	○	○	○	○

11) How TRUE or FALSE is *each* of the following statements for you?

	Definitely true	Mostly true	Don't know	Mostly false	Definitely false
a. I seem to get sick a little easier than other people	O	O	O	O	O
b. I am as healthy as anybody I know	O	O	O	O	O
c. I expect my health to get worse	O	O	O	O	O
d. My health is excellent	O	O	O	O	O

Acknowledgement

This chapter was modified based on a previously published research article from the author who got the permission to reuse the previous article from the publisher.

References

1   Blumenthal JA, Babyak MA, Moore KA, Craighead WE, Herman S, Khatri P, Waugh R, Napolitano MA, Forman LM, Appelbaum M, Doraiswamy PM, Krishnan KR: Effects of exercise training on older patients with manor depression. Arch Intern Med 1999;159:2349–2356.

2   Paluska SA, Schwenk TL: Physical activity and mental health: Current concepts. Sports Med 2000;29:167–180.

3   Vuori I: Exercise and physical health: musculoskeletal health and functional capabilities. Res Q Exerc Sport 1995;66:276–285.

4   Wolf SL, Coogler C, Xu T: Exploring the basis for Tai Chi Chuan as a therapeutic exercise approach. Arch Phys Med Rehabil 1997;78:886–892.

5   Adams TB, Moore MT, Dye J: The relationship between physical activity and mental health in a national sample of college females. Women Health 2000;45:69–85.

6   Hain TC, Fuller L, Weil L, Kotsias J: Effects of tai chi on balance. Arch Otolaryngol Head Neck Surg 1999;125:1191–1195.

7   Ryan AJ: Tai Chi Chuan for mind and body. Physician Sports Med 1974;3:58–61.

8   Delza S: Tai Chi Quan: Body and mind in Harmony. Albany, New York: State University of New York, 1985.

9   Jacobson BH, Chen HC, Cashhel C, Guerrero L: The effects of T'ai Chi Chuan training on balance, kinesthesis sense, and strength. Percept Mot Skills 1997;84:27–33.

10 Jin P: Changes in heart rate, noradrenaline, cortisol and mood during Tai Chi. J Psychosom Res 1989;33:197–206.

11 Liang S, Wu W: Tai Chi Chuan, 24 & 48 Postures with Martial Applications. Jamaica Plain, MA: YMAA Publication Center, 1996.

12 Tse SK, Bailey DM: Tai Chi and postural control in the well elderly. Am Occup Ther 1992;45:295–300.

13 Wolf SL, Barnhart HX, Elllison GL, Coogler CE: The effects of Tai Chi Quan and computerized balance training on postural stability in older subjects, Atlanta FICSIT Group, Frailty and Injuries: Cooperative Studies on Intervention Techniques. Phys Ther 1997;77:371–384.

14 Wang YT, Taylor L, Pearl M, Chang L: Effects of Tai Chi exercise on physical and mental health of college students. Am J Chin Med 2004;32:453–459.

15 Ware JE, Sherbourne CD: The MOS 36-item short-form health survey (SF-36): Conceptual framework and item selection. Med Care 1992;30:473–481.

16   Ware JE, Kosinski M: SF-36 physical & mental health summary scales: A manual for users of version 1, ed 2. Lincoln, Rhode Island, Quality Metric, Inc., 2001.

17   Freeman LW, Lawlis GF: Complementary & Alternative Medicine – A research-based approach. St. Louis, Missouri, Mosby, Inc., 2001.

18   Green SB, Salkind NJ, Akey TM: Using SPSS for Window — Analysis and Understand Data. Upper Saddle River, New Jersey, PrenticeHall Inc., 2000.

Yong 'Tai' Wang, PhD
Director of Biomechanics Research Laboratory
Division of Physical Therapy, Georgia State University
140 Decatur Street, Building: Urban Life, Suite 1279
Atlanta, GA 30303 (USA)
Tel. +1 404 651 3131, Fax +1 404 651 1584, E-Mail ywang2@gsu.edu

Hong Y (ed): Tai Chi Chuan. State of the Art in International Research.
Med Sport Sci. Basel, Karger, 2008, vol 52, pp 146–154

....

Effect of Tai Chi on Depressive Symptoms amongst Chinese Older Patients with Major Depression: The Role of Social Support

Kee-Lee Chou

Sau Po Centre on Ageing, The University of Hong Kong, Hong Kong, SAR, China

Abstract

The objective of this study was to determine whether the effects of Tai Chi training on depressive symptoms in Chinese older patients with depression remained statistically significant after social support was controlled. Fourteen community-dwelling older patients from a psychogeriatric outpatient clinic were randomly assigned to either a 3-month Tai Chi intervention with 36 sessions or a wait-list control. Depression was assessed by the Center for Epidemiological Studies Depression Scale (CES-D), whereas social support was measured by the Lubben Social Network Scale (LSNS). By performing multiple regression analyses, we examined whether the effect of group assignment (Tai Chi and control groups) on five measures of depressive symptoms (i.e. the total scores of the CES-D scale, and scores of all its subscales including symptoms related to somatic, negative affect, interpersonal relation, and well-being) remained significant after controlling for age, gender, education, and LSNS. Results indicate that the beneficial impact of Tai Chi on five measures of depressive symptoms remained significant when we adjusted for age, gender, and education. On the other hand, the effect of our intervention disappeared when changes of social support were controlled for. Social support might be partly responsible for the effect of Tai Chi on depressive symptoms because practicing Tai Chi is a social activity in nature.

Copyright © 2008 S. Karger AG, Basel

As the world becomes more and more globalized, exchanges between the West and the East become more frequent. With the high degree of specialization of health care and the high cost of Western medicine, there is a growing interest in how Eastern traditional medicine can be harmoniously integrated to provide complimentary modes of treatment in areas such as the mental health of older adults. This notion of Eastern and Western medicine complimenting each other is increased by the advocacy of body-mind medicine, which believes in a holistic view (e.g. the mind and the body are not separable) of the human being rather the dualist model. Tai Chi, a Chinese traditional physical exercise, is one possible form of complimentary medicine for mental health problems in Western as well as Asian countries. Although the beneficial effects of physical exercise on mental health has been well demonstrated in the West, few studies have been conducted to test the effectiveness of Tai Chi in the prevention and treatment of depression among Chinese older adults [for exception, see 1] and, to our knowledge, no study has attempted to identify aspects of the psychological mechanisms underlying its effect. This study aimed to fill this knowledge gap by evaluating the role of social support and cognitive capacity in the effect of Tai Chi on depressive symptoms among older patients with clinical depression. This kind of investigation will provide important information so that we can have a better understanding of the role of Tai Chi in mental health. Consequently, the acceptance of the role of Tai Chi in the broader mental health service sector will be greatly enhanced.

Exercise and Mental Health

Although the beneficial effect of physical exercise on physical health is well-known [2], much less attention has been paid to the therapeutic impact of exercise on mental illnesses [3–5]. Exercise indeed plays a therapeutic role in mental health problems and thus can enhance the quality of life for those elderly with mental disorder. In both clinical or nonclinical areas of mental health, there are five important benefits that are associated with the use of exercise: (a) exercise is highly affordable; (b) exercise could be practiced with minimal supervision; (c) exercise provides an alternative option for those who prefer not to use medication or have no access to intensive counseling services; (d) exercise provides additional physical health benefits that other forms of clinical interventions do not, and (e) the negative side effects (e.g. injury or exercise dependence) of exercise are minimal [4].

Depression and Its Treatment in Hong Kong

Hong Kong has one of the highest elderly suicide rates in the world and many cross-sectional studies have already documented the epidemic of depression among local elderly persons. Recent local epidemiological studies have shown the prevalence rate of depression among older people aged over 65 exceeds 30% [1, 6]. In Hong Kong, prescription drugs continue to be the most frequently used treatment for depression although psychotherapy and ECT might also be used. Exercise has not been routinely used in treatment of depression and this might be due to the fact that mental health service practitioners have a dualist tendency to treat the mind and body as separate entities [7]. More recently, a body-and-mind approach to medicine has been advocated as a better therapeutic model in health care services [8], thereby necessitating additional research into this area.

Exercise and Depression

Previous randomized clinical trial studies have shown that vigorous and regular exercise was related to a significant reduction in depression and that the reduction in depression is of the same order as that found in a variety of standard psychotherapeutic treatment [4, 9]. However, inconsistent findings were found when researchers compared the effect of exercise with traditional treatments (e.g. psychotherapy or behavioral intervention) for depression. In their review paper incorporating a wide variety of subjects, North et al. [10] concluded that exercise reduced depression more than relaxation training or engaging in enjoyable activities, but did not produce effects that were different from psychotherapy. However, in studies with only clinically depressed subjects, exercise produced the same effects as psychotherapy, and behavioral interventions (relaxation or mediation) [11, 12] while exercise used in combination with individual psychotherapy, or exercise together with drug therapy, produced the largest effects. Even though Mutrie cautions that the range of psychotherapeutic techniques used in these studies does not always mirror what is considered best practice for depressed patients, i.e. cognitive-behavioral therapy, determining that exercise is at least as effective as more traditional therapies is encouraging, especially considering the time and cost involved with treatment such as psychotherapy. Thus, because exercise is cost-effective it has positive physical health benefits, it is effective in alleviating depression, and it is a viable adjunct or alternative to many of the more traditional depression therapies. Furthermore, any exercise study is enhanced if the participants have a strong empathy towards the type of intervention since this is likely to promote greater compliance during the intervention and habituation after the intervention ceases. Thus traditional Chinese exercises such as Tai Chi are felt to be highly appropriate for this elderly Chinese population.

Mechanism of How Exercise Works

Although different explanations have been proposed, very little is yet known of the mechanism underlying the effect of exercise on depression [13, 14] and it is the major shortcoming in this area of the literature. It is felt that this short-coming contributes to the lack of acceptance by mental health service professionals of the role exercise can play [15]. Therefore, it is important to try and understand how exercise helps treat depression, but unfortunately few studies have attempted to investigate the mechanism by which the effects of exercise are able help explain the psychological basis of depression [14]. This may be compounded by the multifactorial nature of depression and that the various psychological theories of depression might predict that different mechanisms mediate the impact of exercise on depression. Interpersonal theories of depression may suggest mediators including interpersonal relationship, social support, or seeking reassurance [16].

Chinese Traditional Exercises

Previous studies on the relationship between exercise and depression have emphasized Western styles of aerobic exercise, e.g. walking, jogging, cycling [17]. Only a few studies have been conducted to test the relationship between Chinese traditional exercises, such as Tai Chi and depression. Tai Chi is not only the most popular form of physical exercise among Hong Kong elderly people [18], it is also a style of life that promotes the Taoist philosophical values of 'letting go' of struggles and interpersonal conflicts, maintaining a peaceful mind and a sense of harmony, which are congruent with the Chinese traditional aspiration of life fulfillment. Tai Chi, in its physical and exercise form, is a series of individual dance-like movements linked together in a continuous, smooth-flowing sequence. Various studies have found that the beneficial effects of Tai Chi on physical health [19], are comparable to moderate exercise in older adults [20–22]. Furthermore, with its emphasis on enriching the spiritual mind, it is likely that Tai Chi would also contribute to enhanced mental health, which may even surpass the effects of Western style exercises. In fact, previous studies have shown that Tai Chi reduces mood disturbances just after the exercise [23], enhances psychosocial well-being [24], reduces anxiety in frustration [25], and increases life satisfaction and positive affect [26]. In 2003, we conducted a randomized clinical trial to investigate the impact of Tai Chi on older adults with clinical depression and found that the 3-month Tai Chi intervention with 36 sessions resulted in significant reductions in the total scores of the Center for Epidemiological Studies Depression Scale (CES-D), and scores of all its subscales including symptoms related to somatic, negative affect, interpersonal relation, and well-being. In this paper, we examined the effect of this Tai Chi intervention on the indicators of psychological well-being and evaluated whether the impact of Tai Chi on depressive symptoms is mediated by social support.

Method

Participants

Our study population consisted of community-dwelling depressed patients who attended a psychogeriatric outpatient clinic located in Hong Kong. Thirty patients who met our selection criteria were invited and 14 of them agreed to participate in our study. The screening instrument was the Chinese version of the CES-D [27], which has been validated in previous studies [28]. The inclusion criteria were: (1) fulfillment of the DSM-IV diagnostic criteria for either unipolar major or minor depression or dysthymia but the cause of depression was not organic in nature; (2) a CES-D score at or higher than the common cut-off of 16 for diagnosable depression [29]; (3) age 60 years old and above; (4) no involvement in any regular exercise in the past 6 months; (5) no specific medical contraindication to exercise, e.g. unstable cardiac condition or major stroke; (6) preserved physical ability e.g. whether the subject could move his/her limbs in Tai Chi exercise; (7) intact cognition – scores >25 on the Mini-Mental State Examination [30], and (8) willingness to be randomly assigned to any of the two conditions of this research. The mean age of these 14 selected subjects was 72.6 years (SD = 4.2). Half of them were female. Their mean duration of education was 4.6 years (SD = 4.6). 57.1% were married, 35.7% were widowed, and 7.10% were divorced.

Procedures

Informed consent forms were obtained from study participants. A battery of psychological tests and health indicators was administered at the baseline (pretreatment). Included in this test battery was the Chinese version of the 20-item CES-D scale which was used to measure depressive symptoms. Radloff [27] discussed the properties of the scale and its appropriateness for use with community-dwelling older adults in detail. The participants were asked for 20 depressive symptoms that they might have experienced in the 1-week period preceding the interview. The 20 items were scored on a standard 4-point scale from 0 to 3, and the scale or subscales was the unweighted sum of the corresponding items. The Chinese version of the CES-D had been validated in earlier studies [28, 31], and the back translation was used to make sure the meaning of items in CES-D was the same for Hong Kong Chinese elderly and American elderly. Five scores were obtained from the CES-D as follows: the total 20-item scores, the psychological symptoms scores, the somatic symptoms scores, the interpersonal problem scores, and well-being scores [27, 32]. Participants' social support networks were assessed by the Lubben Social Network Scale (LSNS) [33], which is a 10-item measure of five aspects of social networks: family network, friend networks, helping others, confidant relationships (that is, be a confidant or has a confidant), and living arrangements. The scale has been widely used in studies on the Hong Kong Chinese elderly population [34, 35].

One well-trained interviewer who was blinded to the group assignment and study hypothesis collected the self-reported data in a face-to-face format at participants' residence. Subjects were randomly assigned to one of two conditions: Tai Chi training group (n = 7) and the control group (n = 7). The mean for attendance rate in 36 Tai Chi sessions in the Tai Chi group was 95%. In the Tai Chi training condition, participants received a Tai Chi training program in which participants were instructed to engage in three 45-min sessions per week, throughout the 3-month intervention period. The form of Tai Chi we selected was an 18-form Yang's style [36] which is commonly practiced in Hong Kong aged population. Each session consisted of a 10-min warm-up, 25 min of Tai Chi practice, and a 10-min cool-down. All sessions were led by an experienced Tai Chi practitioner who demonstrated the warm-up and cool-down exercises, taught Tai Chi movements, and promoted relaxation, deep breathing, and concentration of the mind. Subjects in the wait-list condition were told that their treatment would be delayed for 3 months, after which they could choose the Tai Chi program. At the end of the treatment and wait-list conditions, i.e. 3 months after the baseline, all subjects were reassessed on the same battery as at pretreatment.

Data Analysis

To assess the changes in depressive symptoms and social support before and after the Tai Chi intervention, we computed the differences in scores of the 20-item CES-D, four subscales of CES-D (somatic, negative affect, interpersonal, and well-being), and LSNS we measured before and after the clinical trial. Then, we performed regression analyses to examine whether the effect of Tai Chi on depressive symptoms remained significant when participants' age, gender, years of education or social support (measured by LSNS) were controlled.

Results

As can be seen in table 1, the effect of group assignment (Tai Chi and control groups) on five measures of depressive symptoms namely the CES-D scale and its four subscales (somatic, negative affect, interpersonal, and well-being) remained significant after we controlled age, gender or education. However, when we adjusted the changes of social support during the clinical trial, the impact of Tai Chi on all measures of depressive symptoms disappeared.

Conclusion

In our previous study, we have shown that Tai Chi has a positive effect on reducing depressive symptoms compared with no treatment in older patients with depression. Tai Chi is equally effective in reducing all four categories of depressive symptoms including somatic symptoms, psychological symptoms, symptoms related to interpersonal relation, and symptoms associated with well-being. Taken together, these findings show that, at least in short-term, Tai Chi reduces a broad range of depressive symptoms in Chinese older patients with depression.

However, it is important understand the mechanism underlying the positive impact of Tai Chi on depressive symptoms. Results of the current study indicate that social support might partly contribute to the beneficial effect of Tai Chi because Tai Chi is a group activity in which practitioners could receive social support from their peers. Other factors potentially contributing to the positive

Table 1. Main effects of group assignment (Tai Chi and control groups) on depression: results of multiple regression analyses (beta)

Changes in CES-D scores					
Predictor variables					
Group assignment	0.82**	0.72**	0.77**	0.79**	0.40
Age		−0.21			
Gender			−0.34*		
Years of education				0.23	
Changes in LSNS					−0.52
Changes in Somatic symptoms subscale scores					
Predictor variables					
Group assignment	0.66*	0.53*	0.63*	0.66*	0.29
Age		−0.27			
Gender			−0.23		
Years of education				0.04	
Changes in LSNS					−0.46
Changes in Negative affect symptoms subscale scores					
Predictor variables					
Group assignment	0.70**	0.58*	0.66**	0.67**	0.36
Age		−0.23			
Gender			−0.25		
Years of education				0.20	
Changes in LSNS					−0.41
Changes in Interpersonal symptoms subscale scores					
Predictor variables					
Group assignment	0.63*	0.50	0.58*	0.61*	0.38
Age		−0.26			
Gender			−0.33		
Years of education				0.19	
Changes in LSNS					−0.31
Changes in Well-being subscale scores					
Predictor variables					
Group assignment	0.64*	0.60*	0.61*	0.60*	0.12
Age		−0.08			
Gender			−0.23		
Years of education				0.35	
Changes in LSNS					−0.65

$*p < 0.05$; $**p < 0.01$.

effects of Tai Chi practice would also be evaluated in the next phase of studies, e.g. self-efficacy, self-concept, physical health, spiritual well-being and attribution style. Given that the aim is to help our elderly population develop a lifestyle of health maintenance, continual practice of Tai Chi is a highly desirable outcome factor. Identifying the factors that may contribute to persistent Tai Chi practice after the intervention compared to other forms of aerobic exercise would also be of further interest.

Group differences emerged in this study even though the statistical power was low. Nonetheless, the small sample size and the absence of attentional control group make these results suggestive only, and future studies should be conducted to replicate the findings with large sample sizes and with the attentional control group. Moreover, it would be interesting to make a direct comparison of the effect on depressive symptoms of Tai Chi with that of other Western aerobic exercise such as brisk walking.

References

1   Chou KL, Chow NWS, Chi I: Leisure participation and its correlates in Hong Kong Chinese older adults. Ageing Soc 2004;24:617–629.
2   US Department of Health and Human Services: Physical activity and health: A report of the Surgeon General. Atlanta, US Department of Health and Human Services, Public Health Service, CDC: National Center for Chronic Disease Prevention and Health Promotion, 1996.
3   Corbin CB, Pangrazi RP: How much physical exercise is enough? JOPERD 1996;67:33–37.
4   Mutrie N: The relationship between physical activity and clinically defined depression; in Biddle SJH, Fox K, Boutcher SH (eds): Physical Activity and Psychological Well-Being, 2000, pp 46–62.
5   Taylor AH: Physical activity anxiety and stress; in Biddle SJH, Fox K, Boutcher SH (eds): Physical Activity and Psychological Well-Being, 2000, pp 10–45.
6   Woo J, Ho SC, Lau J, Yuen YK, Chiu H, Lee HC, Chi I: The prevalence of depressive symptoms and predisposing factors in an elderly Chinese population. Acta Psych Scand 1994;50:746–754.
7   Beesley S, Mutire N: Exercise is beneficial adjunctive treatment in depression. BMJ 1997;315: 1542–1543.
8   Chan CLW: An eastern body-mind-spirit approach: A training manual with one-second techniques. Department of Social Work and Social Administration, The University of Hong Kong.
9   Mather AS, Rodriguez C, Guthrie MF, McHarg AM, Reid IC, McMurdo MET: Effects of exercise on depressive symptoms in older adults with poorly responsive depressive disorder. Br J Psychiat 2002;180:411–415.
10 North TC, McCullagh P, Tran ZV: Effect of exercise on depression. Exerc Sport Sci R 1990;18: 397–415.
11 Craft LL, Landers DM: The effects of exercise on clinical depression and depression resulting from mental illness: A meta-analysis. J Sport Exerc Psy 1998;20:339–357.
12 Mutire N: Healthy body, healthy mind? Psychologist 2002;15:412–413.
13 Dishman RK: Medical psychology in exercise and sport. Med Clin North Am 1985;69:123–143.
14 Brosse AL, Sheets ES, Lett HS, Blumenthal JA: Exercise and the treatment of clinical depression in adults. Sport Med 2002;32:741–760.
15 Hale AS: ABC of mental health: Depression. BMJ 1997;315:43–46.
16 Coyne JC: Toward an interactional description of depression. Psychiat 1976;39:28–40.
17 McAuley E, Katula JA, Blissmer B, Duncan TE: Exercise environment, self-efficacy, and affective responses to acute exercise in older adults. Psychol Health 1999;15:1–15.

18   Cheng YH, Chou KL, MacFarlance DJ, Chi I: Patterns of physical exercise and contributing factors among Hong Kong older adults. Hong Kong Med J 2007;13:S7–S12.
19   Lan C, Lai JS, Chen SY: Tai Chi Chuan: an ancient wisdom in exercise and health promotion. Sport Med 2002;32:217–224.
20   Hartman CA, Manos TM, Winter C: Effects of Tai Chi training on function and quality of life indicatiors in older adults with osteoarthritis. JAGS 2000;48:1553–1559.
21   Li F, Harmer P, McAuley E, Duncan TE, Duncan SC, Chaumeton N, Fisher KJ: An evaluation of the effects of Tai Chi exercise on physical function among older persons: a randomized controlled trial. Ann Behav Med 2001;23:139–146.
22   Choi JH, Moon JS, Song R: Effects of Sun-style Tai Chi exercise on physical fitness and fall prevention in fall-prone older adults. J Adv Nurs 2005;51:150–157.
23   Brown DR, Wang Y, Wade A, Ebbeling CB, Fortage L, Puleo E, Benson H, Rippe JM: Chronic psychological effects of exercise and exercise plus cognitive strategies. Med Sci Sports Exerc 1995;27:765–775.
24   Cheng WK, Macfarlane DJ: Effects of a modified Tai Chi programme on the physical and psychological well-being of elderly Chinese. Paper presented at the 2nd International Symposium on Chinese Elderly, Shanghai, China, 2001.
25   Jin PT: Efficacy of Tai Chi, brisk walking, meditation and reading in reducing mental and emotional stress. J Psychosomat Res 1992;36:361–370.
26   Li F, Duncan TE, Duncan SC, McAuley E, Chaumeton NR, Harmer P: Enhancing the psychological well-being of elderly individuals through Tai Chi exercise: A latent growth curve analysis. Struct Equ Modeling 2001;8:53–83.
27   Radloff LS: The CES-D Scale: a self-report depression scale for research in the general population. Appl Psych Meas 1977;140:385–401.
28   Chi I, Boey KW: Hong Kong validation of measuring instruments of mental health status of the elderly. Clin Gerontol 1993;13:35–51.
29   Lewinsohn PM, Seeley JR, Roberts RE, Allen NB: Center for Epidemiologic Studies Depression Scale (CES-D) as a screening instrument for depression among community-residing older adults. Psychol Ageing 1997;12:277–287.
30   Folstein MF, Folstein SE, McHugh PR: Mini-mental state: a practical method of grading the cognitive state of patients for the clinician. J Psychiat Res 1975;12:189–198.
31   Chi I: Mental health of the old-old in Hong Kong. Clin Gerontol 1995;15:31–44.
32   Sheehan TJ, Fifield J, Reisine S, Tennen H: The measurement structure of the Center for Epidemiological Studies Depression Scale. J Pers Assess 1995;64:507–521.
33   Lubben JE: Assessing social networks among elderly populations. J Fam Community Health 1988;11:45–52.
34   Chou KL, Chi I: Determinants of life satisfaction among Chinese older adults: a longitudinal study. Aging Ment Health 1999;3:327–334.
35   Chou KL, Chi I: Reciprocal relationship between social support and depressive symptoms among Chinese elderly. Aging Ment Health 2003;7:224–231.
36   Chow M: Classical Yang Style Tai Chi Chuan. LA, Wen Lin.

Kee-Lee Chou, BSocSc, MA, PhD
Associate Professor
Department of Social Work and Social Administration
The University of Hong Kong
Pokfulam Road, Hong Kong, SAR (China)
Tel. +852 2241 5940, Fax +852 2858 7604, E-Mail klchou@hku.hk

Hong Y (ed): Tai Chi Chuan. State of the Art in International Research.
Med Sport Sci. Basel, Karger, 2008, vol 52, pp 155–165

....

Tai Chi Exercise and the Improvement of Health and Well-Being in Older Adults

Matthew Kwai-sang Yau

Department of Rehabilitation Sciences, The Hong Kong Polytechnic University,
Hong Kong, SAR, China

Abstract

Activity participation has a positive impact on both quantity and quality of life (QOL).
Regular participations in physical, social, and cultural activities are associated with successful aging. There is considerable evidence that Tai Chi has positive health benefits; physical,
psychosocial and therapeutic. Furthermore, Tai Chi does not only consist of a physical component, but also sociocultural, meditative components that are believed to contribute to overall well-being. This chapter describes the benefits of Tai Chi exercise for the older adults,
particularly in terms of the psychosocial aspect. The perceived meanings, associated values
and well-being, as well as the impact on QOL, of Tai Chi practice among the older adults in
Hong Kong are also discussed. Tai Chi exercise is chosen by the elderly participants for its
gentle and soft movements. Besides the physical aspect, the benefits they describe include
lifestyle issues, as well as psychological and social benefits. Evidence points out that the
improvements in physical and mental health through the practice of Tai Chi among the older
adults are related to their perceived level of QOL. Findings from numerous studies support
the belief that the practice of Tai Chi has multiple benefits to practitioners that are not only
physical in nature. It is recommended as a strategy to promote successful aging.

Copyright © 2008 S. Karger AG, Basel

Meeting the social and health needs of aging population is one of the major
challenges confronting all governments in the 21 century as elderly citizens
become a growing segment in all countries. The United States Census Bureau
projects that by the year 2020, 17.7% of the population will be aged 65 or over
and that this figure will grow to 22.9% in 2050 [1]. Other countries such as
Japan, Germany, France, and the UK are projected to reach these figures 20
years earlier than the US [2]. Hong Kong, for example, has a current population
of 7 million. By the year 2025, it is predicted that 25% of the Hong Kong population will be over the age of 65 [3].

On the other hand, another fact is dominating the gerontological literature. Rowe, a US-based gerontologist points out that there is a 'compression of morbidity' in old age today – more people are living longer but they are also living healthier [4]. The prevalence of many chronic disorders is falling; 89% of those 65–74 (the young old) now report no disability, and 40% of those over 85 (the oldest old) have no functional deficits. Taking the US as example, a 65-year-old American male, on average, can expect to spend 12 of his remaining 15 years fully independent [4].

How the 20–25% of our populations will occupy their time, maintain their health and find meaning during the postretirement years to enhance their well-being is of concern to individuals, families, health care providers and governments. Furthermore, the psychosocial benefits that result from participation in specific activities or types of activities, particularly from the practitioners' perspective, will provide a powerful basis for health promotion at both the individual and community level. This chapter aims to synthesize the current findings, both empirical and qualitative, on the psychosocial benefits of Tai Chi exercise in promoting health and well-being among the older adults.

Successful Aging

Despite the fact that consensus has not been reached regarding the definition of successful aging, there is emerging agreement over many of the components. A low probability of disease and disease-related disability is a primary condition that separates successful aging from pathological or usual aging (nonpathological but with a high risk for ageing processes) [5]. However, other components also are required. These include cognitive and physical/biological function [5]; mental function [6]; life satisfaction [6]; personal control [6], and social/interpersonal relationships and competency [5, 6]. Furthermore, pursuing meaningful and productive activities appear to contribute to both quality of life (QOL) [5] and slowing down the onset of some health risks.

In fact, the World Health Organization launched the revised disablement classification, now called the Classification of Functioning, Disability and Health (ICF) in November of 2001 [7]. The classification provides both a language to describe and investigate issues related to functioning, disability and health as well as a multidirectional model that begins to display the complexity of relationships between health, body functions, activities, participation, personal factors and the environment [7]. It is the relationship between participation and health that is of particular concern when exploring postretirement activity patterns.

Furthermore, engagement in activity has become synonymous with positive or successful ageing. Rowe further maintains that successful aging is more than avoidance or delay of pathology but also includes maintenance or enhancement of physical and cognitive function and full engagement in life, including productive activities and interpersonal relationships [4]. The opposite is also now observed. Lack of participation in activities is considered an indication of less successful aging [8]. The concepts of participation (through self-selected activities, such as Tai Chi exercise), health, and QOL are consistent with the tenets of activity theory [9], which provides a framework for understanding the relationship between participation and health. Those concepts are further explored in the sections below.

Participation and Well-Being

There is abundant evidence to indicate significant relationships between exercise, health and functioning of older adults [10, 11], as well as between exercise and positive mood [12]. Elderly persons who exercise may also experience an enhanced sense of well-being [13]. However, recent research is now showing that 'successful aging' is also strongly correlated with other factors. For example, lifestyle and daily routine, social support mechanisms, autonomy and control each play an important part in maintaining health and independence [14].

Lifestyle and Daily Routine

Daily or regular participation in activities other than exercise has been shown to increase both the quantity and quality of life. Increased life span has been reported in two large prospective studies examining participation in social, productive and cultural activities. A prospective study of 12,982 adults in Sweden concluded that participants who participated in cultural events lived longer than those who rarely attended similar events [15]. A second study by Glass et al. [16] also supports this increased life expectancy. They demonstrated that productive, social and physical activities were each associated with improved mortality rates of 2,761 elderly participants in a 13-year prospective study. In fact, participation in social and/or productive activities that involved little or no enhancement of fitness lowered the risk of all-cause mortality as much as participation in fitness activities.

In addition to increased quantity of life, pursuing meaningful and productive activities and remaining active contribute to QOL [17]. A randomized controlled trial in the United States, examined the benefits of preventive occupational therapy (participation in meaningful activities) as compared to traditional social groups. The results demonstrated significant benefits in terms of health, function and QOL [14]. An interesting feature of this study was the application to a multiethnic sample. When compared to other groups, Asian participants showed greater improvements in life satisfaction, measures of depression and health perceptions [14].

Social Support Mechanisms

As noted above, participation in social activities is associated with increased life span [16]. Social support also contributes to well-being. After controlling for potential confounding effects, the MacArthur studies of successful ageing (n = 1,189 adults of age 70–79) found that respondents with more social ties showed less functional decline [18]. Although participation in physical activity may decline with disability, severity of disability, such as rheumatoid arthritis, does not appear to reduce the level of participation in social activities and people with higher levels of satisfaction with their social network report more positive feelings of well-being [19].

Autonomy and Control

An internal locus of control and/or a sense of perceived control are positively associated with exercise and participation in leisure activities [20] which are in turn linked to greater perceived health and QOL/life satisfaction [20]. Self-selection and choice of activities provides the most meaning and satisfaction for elderly persons, in turn enhancing life satisfaction [21].

Tai Chi Exercise and Older Adults

Tai Chi, also known as Tai Chi Chuan (boxing), is a form of classical Chinese marital art developed 700 years ago. Historically, practicing Tai Chi was to improve or maintain health, ensure self-defense, improve mental accomplishment and to obtain immortality [22]. Adopted by many Chinese as a form of self-strengthening or health maintenance practice, Tai Chi consists of a sequence of 150 movements and postures. Although it is difficult to completely master Tai Chi by ordinary laymen, with perseverance and continuing practice, it is a low cost, safe and enjoyable form of exercise [23]. Often practiced in a group, it also provides an opportunity for socialization [23]. While traditionally, the ultimate goal for learning and practicing Tai Chi was to become immortal, today the popular belief is that it promotes the highest level of longevity [22] as it also provides a vehicle for meditation and spiritual well-being [12].

In Hong Kong and Asia, Tai Chi is particularly popular among older adults due to the gentle movement and the traditional belief that it contributes to 'a happy old age' [24]. Kwan [25], in a review of 17 studies on the needs of the elderly in Hong Kong, reported that besides watching television, Tai Chi and/or 'morning exercise' is the second most popular activity of the elderly and one of the few that is not sedentary. This popularity is not confined to Asia. Studies of Chinese-American elderly adults, who have lived most of their adult lives in the US, show high levels of participation in culturally related activities [26]. Tai Chi is reported as one of the activities which they identify as 'the single activity in which they participate most' [26].

Benefits of Tai Chi Exercise

Despite the fact that Tai Chi has been practiced for hundreds of years, systematic studies of its benefits were not carried out until the late 20th century. These studies, primarily from a medical point of view, have focused on physical, psychological and therapeutic benefits [24]. Since the findings are well documented in other chapters of this book, only the major benefits are recaptured here.

Physical Benefits

The physical benefits of Tai Chi have in fact been extensively investigated [27]. Tai Chi has been shown to increase strength, improve joint flexibility, and relieve muscular tension [24, 28]. Improved balance, posture, and gait are also improved through practice [12, 27]. These in turn have been associated with a reduced risk and fear of falling among the elderly [12, 29]. When practiced by elderly people with motor impairments and/or functional deficits, Tai Chi also appears to lead to improved physical status [23] and lowered risk of falls [30]. Schaller [31] concludes that for all elderly who practice Tai Chi, balance is maintained or improved, but for those elderly adults with some degree of impaired function, it may be even more effective in improving balance.

Psychological Benefits

Tai Chi also has an impact on mental health [29] and is an effective therapeutic tool for stress management. It has been reported to lead to an increase in awareness of somatic tension [12], resulting in reduced anxiety and mood disturbance [22, 32], and an improved ability to focus and concentrate [33]. High levels of tranquility [34], stress reduction and mental relaxation are the reported results [35].

Therapeutic Benefits

In addition to physical and psychological benefits, studies report on the therapeutic and medical benefits of Tai Chi. Relief from symptoms of pain and insomnia are often reported [29] as are improvements related to a number of diseases including rheumatoid arthritis, osteoarthritis and osteoporosis [24]; chronic pulmonary disease [24]; depression and chronic fatigue syndrome [24]. Improvement of cardiovascular fitness [36] and enhancement of immunity in older people [37] may contribute, in part to the reported therapeutic benefits. In a quasi-experimental study (n = 39), Taylor-Piliae et al. [32] further found in their 12-week Tai Chi exercise program for older adult immigrants of Chinese background that the exercise statistically significantly increased subjects' self-efficacy to overcome barriers to Tai Chi, confidence to perform the exercise, and perceived social support.

A Study on the Meanings and Perceived Benefits of Tai Chi among the Older Adults

To add to the objective findings on the benefits of Tai Chi as mentioned above, a descriptive study was conducted by Yau and Packer [38] to gain an in-depth understanding of the perceived importance, meanings and health benefits from the perspective of a group of elderly, long-term Tai Chi practitioners in Hong Kong. In addition, the participants' perspective on Tai Chi and its contribution to QOL were explored.

Methodology

This study, adopting a qualitative approach employing focus group techniques, explored the perceived importance, meanings, and health benefits of participation in Tai Chi by people over the age of 55 in Hong Kong. Purposive sampling was used to recruit informants for focus groups to explore the topic in depth [39]. Participants provide an audience for one another that encourages discussion such that information including a wide range of opinions, attitudes, and behaviors can be collected.

Subjects

Regular Tai Chi practitioners were contacted through Tai Chi masters and invited to participate. Four focus groups were formed with a total of 18 participants; the number of participants in each group ranged from 3 to 6. In one group, 3 participants had visible physical disabilities; they too were regular practitioners of Tai Chi. Participants ranged in age from 51 to 85 years with a mean age of 67. The average years practicing Tai Chi was 8.5 years (range 3–26) with more than two thirds of the participants practicing Tai Chi daily for at least 1 hour.

Data Collection and Analysis

Each focus group, moderated by a trained research assistant, lasted 1–1.5 hour, and was conducted in Cantonese, the common local dialect. A focus-group guide was developed based on the literature and key informant information. Although a number of core questions were predesigned and asked, additional questions were developed on the spot for clarification and elaboration of any arising themes.

All focus groups were audio-taped and subsequently transcribed and coded using constant comparative method. Two researchers independently coded the transcripts using content analysis to identify common themes in the responses of the participants, as well as to increase the credibility and trustworthiness of the data.

Findings

Two recurring themes echo throughout the data: participation provides meaning and a pattern to daily life, and participation promotes health and well-being. Each theme is described in more detail below, as well as the perceived relationship between Tai Chi and QOL.

Participation Provides Meaning and Pattern to Life
Participants in the focus groups were all long-term practitioners of Tai Chi. It is, therefore, not surprising that Tai Chi formed part of their daily routine.

However, the extent to which Tai Chi became a focus around which they organized their day was noteworthy. Analysis indicated that two main ideas domi-
nated their perceptions about participation in Tai Chi: firstly, they consistently
reported that the characteristics of Tai Chi were a 'good fit' for older adults. It is
described as 'soft', 'less vigorous with gentle movements', 'effortless' and 'in
slow motion'. These qualities also provided their rationale for recommending
Tai Chi as opposed to other activities.

Secondly, that regular practice of Tai Chi carried over into other aspects of
their daily routine such that it created a comfortable rhythm and pattern in daily
life. The early morning practice of Tai Chi set the tone of the day, provided a
temporal reference and appeared to provide a focal point for planning. This
morning routine was credited with benefits throughout the rhythm of the day at
home, work and within the family. The importance of this 'anchor' to the day
appeared to be important both for those who still work, as well as those who are
retired.

Participation Leads to Health and Well-Being

Participation in Tai Chi provides a strong source of mutual social support
and encourages development of inner calmness, both highly valued but intangi-
ble assets of participation. The positive atmosphere of practicing in groups was
highly valued by participants. This positive atmosphere promoted strong mutual
support that went beyond the time designated for participation. The mutual
support extended to companionship, concern for each other, and sharing of
experiences.

More directly, participants also strongly perceived Tai Chi as an active
strategy to improve physical and mental health. Many participants directly
related health benefits to participation in Tai Chi; physical, cognitive and mental health benefits. Accompanying this improved health was a new belief in
their ability to take active control of their health with positive results.

Perceived Relationship between Tai Chi and QOL

Despite the fact that QOL is not a familiar term or concept for elderly
adults in Hong Kong, after clarification with examples by the researchers, the
participants seemed to be able to relate the practice of Tai Chi to their understanding of QOL. They perceived these improved physical, psychological,
social and lifestyle benefits, to be linked to improved QOL. It was interesting
that the psychological, social and lifestyle benefits were more strongly linked to
QOL than the physical benefits. Specifically, improvement in marital relationships, memory and cognitive function, mental alertness, stress management,
and temperament and outlook were highlighted as important. In particular,
many participants found that they were able to control their emotions and

maintain calmness to deal with life's problems. Furthermore, as the participants were all devoted practitioners, their responses might have been skewed. However, a search of the literature also failed to find any significant negative effects or contraindications for the Tai Chi exercise.

Conclusion

Activity participation has a positive impact on both quantity and quality of life. Regular participations in physical, social, and cultural activities are associated with successful aging. Autonomy, perceived control and social support networks are now believed to be key factors. There is considerable evidence that Tai Chi has physical, psychosocial and therapeutic health benefits. Tai Chi has both a physical component as well as a sociocultural, meditative component that is believed to contribute to overall well-being.

Studies also indicate that Tai Chi is considered a smooth, gentle and soft exercise. Although it is suitable for all ages, elderly adults feel it suits their needs for safety, has limited barriers and is matched to their ability level. The perceived benefits that accrue from participation include: (1) participation provides meaning and pattern to life, and (2) participation leads to health and well-being. These benefits often extend to family, work and daily interactions. The findings from the numerous studies have further supported the idea that the practice of Tai Chi has multiple benefits, and due to its reduced physical demand, Tai Chi may provide an excellent strategy for health promotion and successful aging.

References

1   Angel JL, Hogan DP: The demography of minority aging populations. J Fam Hist 1992;17:95–116.
2   Anderson GF, Hussey PS: Datawatch: Population Aging: a comparison among individualized countries; populations around the world are growing older, but the trends are not cause for despair. Health Aff 2000;19:191–204.
3   Philips DR: Experiences and implications of demographics aging in the Asia-Pacific. Hong Kong J Gerontol 1995;9:20–29.
4   Rowe JW: The new gerontology. Science 1997;278:367–370.
5   Rowe J, Kahn R: Successful aging. Gerontologist 1997;37:433–440.
6   Baltes PB, Baltes MM: Psychological perspectives on successful aging: The model of selective optimization with compensation; in Baltes PB, Baltes MM (eds): Successful aging. Cambridge, England: Cambridge University Press, 1990, pp 1–34.
7   World Health Organization: International classification of functioning, disability and health 2000 Retrieved April 4, 2002 from the World Wide Web: http://www.who.int/classification/icf/intros/ICF-Eng-Intro.pdf.
8   Horgas AL, Wilms HU, Baltes MM: Daily life in very old age: everyday activities as expression of successful living. Gerontologist 1998;38:556–568.

9   McIntosh BR, Danigelis NL: Race, gender, and the relevance of productive activity for elders' affect. J Gerontol Soc Sci 1995;50B:S229–S239.

10 Blair SN, Garcia ME: Get up and move: A call to action for older men and women. J Am Geriatr Soc 1996;44:599–600.

11 Ettinger WH Jr: Physical activity and older people: A walk a day keeps the doctor away. J Am Geriatr Soc 1996;44:207–208.

12 Sandlund ES, Norlander T: The effects of tai chi chuan relaxation and exercise on stress responses and well-being: an overview of research. Int J Stress Manage 2000;7:139–149.

13 Zimmer L, Lin HS: Leisure activity and well-being among the elderly in Taiwan: Testing hypothesis in an Asian setting. J Cross Cult Gerontol 1996;11:167–186.

14 Clark F, Azen SP, Zemke R, Jackson J, Carlson M, Mandel D, Hay J, Josephson K, Chery B, Hessel C, Palmer J, Lipson L: Occupational therapy for independently-living older adults. JAMA 1997;279:1321–1326.

15 Bygren LO, Konlaan BB, Johansson SE: Attendance at cultural events, reading books or periodicals, and making music or singing in a choir as determinants for survival: Swedish interview survey of living conditions. BMJ 1996;313:1577–1580.

16 Glass TA, de Leon CM, Marottoli RA, Berkman LF: Population based study of social and productive activities as predictors of survival among elderly American. BMJ 1999;319:478–484.

17 Fisher BJ: Successful aging, life satisfaction, and generativity in later life. Int J Aging Hum Dev 1995;41:239–250.

18 Unger JB, McAvay G, Bruce ML, Berkman L, Seeman T: Variation in the impact of social network characteristics on physical functioning in elderly persons: MacArthus studies of successful aging. J Gerontol B Psychol Sci Soc Sci 1999;54B:S245–S251.

19 Zimmer Z, Hickey T, Serale MS: Activity participation and well-being among older people with arthritis. Gerontologist 1995;35:463–471.

20 Menec VA, Chipperfield JG: Remaining active in later life: The role of locus of control in seniors' lecture activity participation, health and life satisfaction. J Aging Health 1997;9:105–125.

21 Beard JG, Ragheb MG: Measuring leisure satisfaction. J Leisure Res 1980;12:20–33.

22 Olson SA: Tai Chi Chuan. Minnesota: D.W. Friesen & Sons Ltd, 1984.

23 Wolf SL, Coolger C, Xu T: Exploring the basis for Tai Chi Chuan as a therapeutic exercise approach. Arch Phys Med 1997;78:886–892.

24 Ross MC, Preswalla JL: The therapeutic effects of tai chi for the elderly. J Gerontol Nurs 1998;24:45–47.

25 Kwan AYH: A review of the recreation and leisure activities patterns of older people in Hong Kong, 1972–1990. Hong Kong J Gerontol 1990;4:28–34.

26 Allison MT, Geiger CW: Nature of leisure activities among the Chinese-American elderly. Leisure Sci 1993;15:309–319.

27 Li JX, Hong Y, Chan KM: Tai chi: physiological characteristics and beneficial effects on health. Br J Sport Med 2001;35:148–156.

28 Wolfson L, Whipple R, Derby C, Judge J, King M, Amerman P, Schmidt J, Smyers D: Balance and strength training in older adults: intervention gains and Tai Chi maintenance. J Am Geriatr Soc 1996;44:599–600.

29 Cerrato P: Tai Chi: a martial art turns therapeutic. RN 1999;62:59–60.

30 Zeeuwe P, Verhagen A, Bierma-Zeinstra S, van Rossum E, Faber MJ, Koes B: The effect of Tai Chi Chuan in reducing falls among elderly people: design of a randomized clinical trial in the Netherlands. BMC Geriatrics 2006;6:6.

31 Schaller KJ: Tai Chi Chih-an exercise option for older adults. J Gerontol Nurs 1996;22:12–17.

32 Taylor-Piliae RE, Haskell W, Waters C, Froelicher ES: Change in perceived psychosocial status following a 12-week Tai Chi exercise programme. J Adv Nurs 2006;54:313–329.

33 Kutner NG, Barnhart H, Wolf SL, McNeely E, Xu T: Self-report benefits of Tai Chi practice by older adults. J Gerontol Nurs 1997;52:1–6.

34 Szabo A, Mesko A, Caputo A, Gill ET: Examination of exercise-induced feeling states in four modes of exercise. Int J Sports Psychol 1999;29:376–390.

35 Jin P: Changes in heart rate, noradrenaline, cortisol and mood during Tai Chi. J Psychosom Res 1989;33:197–206.

36   Downing JH, Yan J: Tai Chi: an alternative exercise form for seniors. J Aging Phys Activ 1998;6: 350–362.
37   Xusheng S, Yugi X, Ronggang Z: Detection of ZC rosette-forming lymphocytes in the healthy aged with Taichiquan (88 style) exercise. J Sport Med Phys Fit 1990;30:401–405.
38   Yau MK, Packer TL: Health and Well-being through T'ai Chi: Perceptions of Older Adults in Hong Kong. Leisure S 2002;21:163–178.
39   Phan TT, Fitzgerald MH: Guide for the use of focus groups in health research. Sydney: Transcultural Mental Health Center, 1996.

Matthew Kwai-sang Yau, BAppSc, MCom, MSc(Hons), PhD, OTR, CST
Department of Rehabilitation Sciences, The Hong Kong Polytechnic University
Hung Hom, Hong Kong (China)
Tel. +852 2766 6751, Fax +852 2330 8656, E-Mail Matthew.Yau@polyu.edu.hk

Hong Y (ed): Tai Chi Chuan. State of the Art in International Research.
Med Sport Sci. Basel, Karger, 2008, vol 52, pp 166–172

....

Teaching Tai Chi with Mindfulness-Based Stress Reduction to Middle School Children in the Inner City: A Review of the Literature and Approaches

Robert B. Wall

MGH Institute of Health Professions, and Uphams Corner Health Center, Boston, Mass., USA

Abstract

Tai Chi (TC) is the focus of a growing body of literature both qualitative and empirical. Yet there is a paucity of literature on teaching TC to either adolescents or children ages 10–13 presumably because of the level of attention and concentration TC requires. In the pediatric setting, TC appears best combined with other practice activities like mindfulness-based stress reduction (MBSR) that complement the practice of TC, sustain interest and synergistically enhance the benefits TC has been shown to produce in older populations. The literature on the effects of (MBSR) practices with children and teens are also limited. However, the corpus of TC studies suggests significant benefits could be transgenerational if presented in novel ways and taught in developmentally appropriate approaches to children. This chapter explores combining MBSR exercises with TC as one practice that can potentially accomplish this synergy. The chapter includes recommendations for a course design based on two projects created by the author integrating TC and MBSR for ages 11–14 in the inner city of Boston, Mass., USA.

Tai Chi (TC) is the focus of a growing body of literature both qualitative and empirical. TC has its origins in antiquity and grew out of shamanistic dances patterned after animals [1]. Forms of these patterns come down to us now in varied and widely performed health promotion activity called chi kung or qi gong [1, 2]. The TC movements encourage sensitivity to internal sensation and demand concentration and attention and as such are recommended for health promotion in adults. This chapter reviews selected literature and explores the social question of whether and how TC can be taught to children at middle school age 11–13.

A Review of Selected Literature: Can TC Be Taught to Children?

Searching Tai Chi and Tai Ji using search engines such as the Cumulative Index of Nursing and Allied Health Literature, Ovid Medline, and other nonindexed citations from 1950 to the present yielded 1,186 citations. The vast foci of these citations were on the use of TC in older adults. Only two citations from this search were focused directly on the impact of TC on children [3, 4]. One reason supposed for the lack of studies of TC with children and adolescents is the increased demand TC places on the student for attention, concentration, precision and the slowness required to execute the movements exactly. Traditionally, because of their age, TC has not been easily taught to children ages 11–14. This has undoubtedly discouraged research into TC in the pediatric population, and is one explanation of the paucity of literature on the subject. However, the corpus of studies suggests significant benefits could be transgenerational if presented in novel ways and taught in developmentally appropriate approaches to children.

The two articles on TC, specific to children, show that TC can be taught to young populations with self-reported positive attitudes toward TC practice, and when combined with other activities result in socially positive outcomes.

Baron [3] examined the psychological effects (self-competence, visual-motor integration, reduction in anxiety) of a TC class for fourth to sixth graders (ages 10–12). After pre-testing, students were randomly assigned to an experimental group for a 12-week TC program, or to a comparison group following usual school routines. Results found that the experimental TC group did not demonstrate improved perceived self-competence, visual-motor integration, or reduced trait anxiety. However, self-reports indicated very positive attitudes toward TC practice.

This writer used a novel approach teaching TC to two groups of 6th grade girls and 8th grade boys aged 11–13 in a Boston public middle-school that integrated TC with mindfulness-based stress reduction exercises (MBSR) [4]. During and after the program, students reported subjective statements of well-being, calmness, relaxation, improved sleep, less reactivity, increased self-care, self-awareness, and a sense of interconnection or interdependence with nature [4].

In the popular literature, searched on Amazon.com, only a few books were published on TC for children. Each integrates TC practices or TC-like movements with other practices to create fun ways for children to learn to play with their posture and movement in Tai-Chi-like-ways that promote a holistic experience.

In view of this literature on TC in the pediatric population, TC can be taught to children; however, it appears best when combined with other practice activities in order to sustain interest and synergistically enhance the benefits that TC practice produces in other populations. This chapter considers MBSR as one such practice that can potentially accomplish this synergy with TC in the pediatric population.

MBSR, like TC, has been widely studied in adults. MBSR was so named and developed by Kabat-Zinn and colleagues at the University of Massachusetts Medical Center, and was taught through a variety of exercises and methods presented systematically in an 8-week educational format [5]. The methods were designed to engender mindfulness.

Mindfulness can be defined as a nonjudgmental attention to all stimuli that emerge into one's field of awareness on a moment-by-moment basis. The stance is one of compassion, befriending, interest and openness toward experience whether pleasant or unpleasant [6]. The MBSR program is premised on the thesis that engendering nonjudgmental awareness to real-time experience helps one disengage from self-related thoughts, feelings, and perceptions that can have a detrimental impact (e.g. anxiety) on the person [5, 6].

A Review of Selected Literature on MBSR: What Is Its Effect on Children?

Selected studies show MBSR, like TC, conferring health benefits on adult populations. Diverse examples include studies using meditation with cancer patients [7], promoting health in inner city bilingual populations [8], to evidence correlating increased neural changes in the brains of adult meditators in cortical areas known to mediate emotional regulation [9, 10].

The literature on the effects of mindfulness with children and teens is more robust than on TC [8, 11–17].

Ott [11, 12] showed that mindfulness practice could easily be taught to children in combination with yoga or by itself to produce positive outcomes.

Semple et al. [13] found preliminary support for treating childhood anxiety in a small sample of 7–8 year olds with group mindfulness techniques. Following this, they reported significantly reduced attentional problems in 9- to 12-year-olds exposed to a 12-week manualized protocol using MBSR [14]. Participants who completed the program showed trends of lessening anxiety and depressive symptoms. The researchers found that all children in the study easily understood the mindfulness concepts being taught, participated readily in activities using various senses, and involved themselves in finding ways to apply their new knowledge to everyday situations. Parental ratings were also positive citing improvements in academic performance and regulating formerly problematic behaviors.

Bootzin and Stevens [15] used MBSR in an integrated approach teaching sleep hygiene in adolescents with substance abuse history and sleep disturbance because insomnia is highly correlated with recidivism. They found those students who completed at least four sessions of an eight-session manualized program had improved sleep and less risk of recidivism.

MBSR practices have profound consequences for reducing morbidity in adolescence into adulthood through methods that address emotional regulation and increase tolerance of stress [8, 16]. An example of a successful clinical intervention using MBSR is called dialectical behavior therapy, which teaches emotional regulation to parasuicidal, stress-intolerant youth [17].

Self-Regulation as the Basis for Learning

Self-regulation of emotion and attention is a prerequisite for both children and adults in order for learning to occur [14]. Learning is supported by a safe holding environment and reliable structure that children need [18]. Learning is enhanced by acquiring skills that help children regulate their emotions with an enhanced sense of self-awareness. Diekman found that the domain of self-awareness is present in children and should be considered to be constant throughout the life cycle. He suggested that practices like mindfulness increase our capacity to respond to experience consciously, providing us with a greater range of conscious choice while reducing emotional reactivity to experience [see 14].

To summarize, mindfulness practices with adolescents teaches emotional regulation skills that promote self-care, and provide a protective factor reducing the risk of longer-term maladaptive development. The data suggest that when combined, MBSR and TC have the potential to help the student regulate emotional reactivity, interest students, and provide concrete strategies for adolescents and children to contain emotionally laden stress.

Elements for Designing a TC/MBSR Program for Children

In response to the child's need for structure, teaching TC/MBSR should include some ground rules that are not usually needed when teaching adults [14]. These include valuing kindness in actions and speech, not talking when another is speaking, raising one's hand 'to get the floor', sharing ideas with the group, not talking during mindfulness exercises, and creating an option to sit out of an exercise (in a designated quiet space).

Designing a TC program for children should consider the following recommendations.

Mastery of TC by the facilitator is not necessary but there should be a working command of the simple elements outlined below. It is appropriate to team teach MBSR and TC; however, MBSR must be practiced by both facilitators because it is essential in order to replace another skill set (didactic model/goal oriented) with a new set of skills that emphasize nonjudgment and acceptance over quantitative change.

The program should be located in a school where children, parents and/or faculty are located at school and can be engaged [14, 19].

Group teaching is preferred over individual training. Through group sharing adolescent students learn from each other and become aware of their own idiosyncratic perceptual 'filters'. MBSR emphasizes developing nonjudgmental language that describes the interaction of thoughts, feeling and bodily sensations and how they influence behavior in real-time situations [14].

Core to children's learning and practicing is establishing a working relationship with the parents around the techniques being learned using homework that can be done in exercises of about 10–15 min [14].

A course design is suggested here. Each session can be 60–90 min (adult classes are 2 h) [4]. The six TC elements simplified from the Yang Style Form are Wu Chi/Opening TC, Grasping Bird's Tail, Ward Off, Two Hand Press, Two Hand Push, and Closing TC Hun Yuan stance [4, 20]. MBSR exercises are included [4, 5].

Suggested course design, TC and MBSR:

Week 1
- Introduction to TC.
- Introductions among group members, group process, expectations for participation.
- Brief discussion of TC as an approach to stress reduction.
- Abdominal breathing seated, lying down, standing [5, p. 72; 20, pp. 54–60].
- Body scan [5, p. 92].

Week 2
- Standing: Iron Shirt lower structure [21, pp. 92–95; 4].
- Standing: Iron Shirt upper structure [21, pp. 96–103; 4].
- Sitting with Breath [5, p. 73; 4].

Week 3
- Standing: Iron Shirt the Rooting Form [21, p. 101].

- Opening TC Form [20, p. 57; 4].
- Breathing, sitting with body as a whole [5, p. 73; 4].
  Week 4
- Opening TC form; Grasping Birds Tail [20, pp. 58–59].
- Two Hand Press [20, pp. 62–62].
- Breathing, Sitting with sound [5, p. 73].
  Week 5
- Wu Chi stance; Opening TC Form; Grasping Birds Tail; Two Hand Press [20, pp. 55–58].
- Two Hand Push [20, p. 63].
- Walking Meditation [5, pp. 114–119; 20, pp. 98–99].
  Week 6
- Wu Chi, Opening TC Form; Grasping Birds Tail; Two Hand Press;
- Two Hand Push.
- Closing TC Hun Yuan stance [20, pp. 80–81; 4].
- Penetrating the unknown: sitting with choiceless awareness [5, p. 74].
  Week 7
- Review.
- Closure.

References

1   Cohen KS: The way of Qigong: The art and science of Chinese energy healing. Ballantine, 1997, pp 12–29.
2   Eisenberg DM, Kessler RC, Foster C, Norlock FE, Calkins DR, Delbanco TL: Unconventional medicine in the United States: Prevalence, costs, and patterns of use. N Engl J Med 1993;328: 246–252.
3   Baron L: Tai Chi Practice in the Elementary Classroom. Can J Rsch Early Chlhd Ed 1998;6: 341–352.
4   Wall R: Tai chi and mindfulness-based stress reduction in a Boston public middle school. J Ped HC 2005;19:230–237.
5   Kabat-Zinn J: Full Catastrophe Living: Using the wisdom of your body and mind to face stress, pain, and illness, ed 2. Random House Bantam Dell, 1990, pp 1–14.
6   Kabat-Zinn J: Mindfulness-based interventions in context: Past present, and future. Clin Psy Sic Prac 2003;10:144–156.
7   Speca M, Carlson LE, Goddey E, Angen M: A randomized, wait-list controlled clinical trial: The effects of a mindfulness meditation-based stress reduction program on mood and symptoms of stress in cancer patients. Am Psyc Som Med 2000;62:613–622.
8   Roth B, Robbins D: Mindfulness-based stress reduction and health-related quality of life: Findings from a bilingual inner-city patient population. Psyc Som Med 2004,66:113–123.
9   Lazar SW, Kerr CE, Wasserman RH, Gray JR, Greve DN, Treadway MT, et al: Meditation experience is associated with increased cortical thickness. NeuroReport 2005;16:1893–1897.
10 Lazar SW, Bush G, Gollub RL, Fricchione GL, Khalsa G, Benson H: Functional brain mapping of the relaxation response and meditation. NeuroReport 2000;11:1581–1585.
11 Ott MJ: Mindfulness meditation in pediatric clinical practice. Pediatr Nurs 2002;28:487–491.
12 Ott MJ: Yoga as a clinical intervention. Adv Nurse Pract 2002;10:81–84.

13   Semple RJ, Reid EFG, Miller L: Treating anxiety with mindfulness: An open trial of mindfulness training for anxious children. J Cog Psy 2005;19:387–400.
14   Semple RJ, Lee J, Miller LF: Mindfulness-Based cognitive therapy for children; in Baer RA (ed): Mindfulness-Based Treatment Approaches: Clinician's guide to evidence base and applications. Elsevier, 2006, pp 143–164.
15   Bootzin RR, Stevens SJ: Adolescents, substance abuse, and the treatment of insomnia and daytime sleepiness. Cl Psyc Rev 2005;25:629–644.
16   Cooper LM, Wood PK, Orcutt HK, Albino A: Personality and the predisposition to engage in risky or problem behaviors during adolescence. J Pers Soc Psy 2003;82:390–410.
17   Wagner EE, Rathus JH, Miller AL: Mindfulness in dialectical behavior therapy (DBT) for adolescents; in Baer RA (ed): Mindfulness-Based Treatment Approaches: Clinician's guide to evidence base and applications. Elsevier, 2006, pp 174–176.
18   Bion W: Attacks on linking. Int J Psychanl 1959;303–315; in Twemlow SW, Fonagy P, Sacco FC: Feeling safe in school. Smith Coll Stud Soc Wk, 2002, vol 72, pp 303–326.
19   Chen DL, Sherman CP: Teaching balance with tai chi: Strategies for college and secondary school instruction. J Phy Ed Rec Dnc 2002;73:31–37, 57.
20   Chia M, Li J: The inner structure of Tai Chi. Healing Tao Books, 1996, pp 55–81.
21   Chia M: Iron Shirt Chi Kung I. Healing Tao Books, 1986, pp 87–111.

Robert B. Wall, M.Div., MSN, FNP-BC, CNS
Family Nurse Practitioner
Psychiatric Nurse Practitioner
13 Crombie Street
Salem, MA 01970 (USA)
Tel. +1 617 740 8066, Fax +1 617 282 7603, E-Mail rwall@partners.org

Hong Y (ed): Tai Chi Chuan. State of the Art in International Research.
Med Sport Sci. Basel, Karger, 2008, vol 52, pp 173–181

....

Tai Chi Chuan in the Management of Parkinson's Disease and Alzheimer's Disease

Penelope J. Klein

D'Youville College, Buffalo, N.Y., USA

Abstract

Background: Parkinson's disease (PD) and Alzheimer's disease (ALZ) represent later-life onset neurodegenerative disorders that gradually rob those afflicted of their quality of life. **Purpose:** This chapter offers practice-based recommendations on how instruction and practice of Tai Chi Chuan (TCC) can be adapted for individuals with PD and those with ALZ. **Research Evidence:** Practice of TCC is widely advocated as an exercise option in PD; however, little validating research exists. Even less is known about feasibility of applications of TCC for individuals with ALZ. **Clinical Impressions:** The slow, rhythmic pace of functionally based exercises, internal organ stimulation, flexibility maintenance, balance-training effects, and general health benefits of TCC and Tai Chi-like exercise practice have clinical relevance for both conditions. Falls prevention, tremor reduction and motor control may be of most importance in management of PD. Behavioral and general health benefits as well as slowing of functional and cognitive decline are considerations with ALZ. **Recommendations:** Strategies of exercise adaptation include use of Tai Chi-like exercise for individuals with ALZ and those in middle or late stages of PD as well as providing instructional resources and training for caregivers and exercise aides to facilitate practice as a part of daily life.

Parkinson's disease (PD) and Alzheimer's disease (ALZ) represent later-life onset neurodegenerative disorders that gradually rob those afflicted of their quality of life. In modern Western medicine, the two pathologies are classified as distinct brain disorders. Cardinal symptoms of PD are tremor, muscular rigidity, bradykinesis, and gait and balance impairment [1].

ALZ is initially experienced as forgetfulness and progresses to profound cognitive impairment manifest as an inability to perform the most basic activities of daily living [2]. Quality of life and caregiving is further challenged by behavioral disorders which are common in later stages of the disease. These include confusion, agitation, depression, aggressiveness and restlessness.

The two clinical conditions are addressed together in this chapter because progressing functional limitations associated with each disorder result in a gradual loss of the ability to complete many basic tasks of daily life, and in both conditions a collaborative management approach is advocated to ensure optimal quality of life and minimization of burden of care through disease progression [3].

The purpose of this chapter is to (a) assess the strength of research evidence assessing whether the practice of Tai Chi Chuan (TCC) might hold any specific benefit for individuals with either PD or ALZ, (b) suggest possible theoretical basis for use of TCC in the management of these disorders, and (c) recommend how instruction and practice of TCC may be adapted for the two clinical populations.

Methods

Methods used included a synthesis of available research and clinical impressions. The search of the literature was conducted through June and July 2007. Key words for intervention included tai chi chuan, taiji, t'ai chi chuh, mind body exercise, Parkinson's disease, Alzheimer's disease, and dementia. Search strategies included use of primary electronic search of PubMed, CINAHL (Ovid), CINAHL (Ebsco) and AMED as well as a search of bibliographic references and Internet sources including public media. Clinical impressions were generated from reflective analysis of published descriptions of model programming and the experiences of the author.

TCC and PD: Research Evidence

There appears to be practice consensus that TCC can be adapted for clinical populations [4] and is an exercise option that may hold specific benefits for individuals with PD [5–7]. However, research studies assessing effect of TCC for individuals with PD are limited. One randomized clinical trial (n = 30) assessed effects of a 12-week program finding falls reduction and slowing of decline of function in those individuals in the Tai Chi group [8]. Two recently published cohort studies offer confirmation of potential benefits. Li et al. [9] assessed effect of a short, 5-day, 90-min per day training program of Tai Chi-based exercises for individuals with mild to moderate PD (n = 17).

On postintervention evaluation, positive effect was observed in functional measures of balance, mobility, and participant satisfaction.

In a one group study, Klein and Rivers [10] explored effects of community TCC group programming for individuals with PD (n = 8) and their support partners (n = 7). On follow-up program evaluation, class participants reported perceiving benefits in physical, emotional and social domains. Improved balance was the most frequently reported physical benefit for individuals with PD. The following study excerpts describe mode and motivation for personal adoption of exercise by individuals with PD:

'I started doing some exercises first thing in the morning to get going' [10, p 24].

'Now, I sometimes do a few minutes of exercising during the day if I feel I am tiring or getting stiff – especially the arm swinging and the breathing' [10, p 24].

'First and foremost – I have found that when my hand shakes, I can stop it by rubbing my hands together and making a small ball to find my chi. This gives me back control. Second – I breath [breathe] deeper, etc, now that I take Tai Chi. Third – Balance is greatly improved' [10, p 26].

Additional empirical evidence of similar experiences with TCC practice by individuals with PD exists as published case study reports [11, 12] and as cited within secondary sources [13].

TCC and PD: Clinical Impressions

Increasing frequency of falls is a diagnostic indicator of advancing PD [14]. There is evidence that TCC training can improve ankle-righting response in individuals with a history of falls [15]. How the influence of TCC practice on ankle righting response might generalize to individuals with PD is a topic for future research.

The elements of continuous movement, slow, reversing movements, synergistic patterns, training in breath regulation and mind-body connection inherent within the art form of TCC distinguish it from other more conventional exercise options such as walking and aerobic circuit training. Basic Tai Chi postures have movement elements similar in pattern and rhythm to slow reversing techniques and movement patterns introduced into conventional physiotherapeutic practice as described by Knott and Voss [16] intended to influence abnormal muscular tone. The slow pacing of TCC exercise may allow time for muscle recruitment within stabilizing muscles and slower twitch fibers of prime movers for strength training and improved coordination of movement. The dynamic quality, body part connectedness, and mental intention of practice may develop kinesthetic awareness and proprioception.

Table 1 describes practice-based recommendations for adapting TCC classes for individuals with PD. These include:

- use of repeated arm swinging as a possible mechanism to release trunk rigidity as a routine preparatory exercise and to offer a visceral massage;
- increase time practicing dynamic balance challenges to include Tai Chi walking and repetitions of backwards walking ('repulse monkey') as well as pivoting and stepping change of direction strategies for falls prevention;
- use reaching movement repetitions such as 'picking fruit' to maintain shoulder flexibility, emphasize awareness of body position in space and 'connectedness' of movements, breathing regulation and calming internal focus for maintaining physical functioning;
- invite family members as caregivers to join in TCC play, and
- provide time for socialization.

TCC and ALZ: Research Evidence

There is epidemiological evidence that regular physical activity is positively associated with reducing cognitive decline in older adults [17]. Exercise is recommended in management of dementia [18]. Regular exercise has been associated with reduced decline of activities of daily living in nursing home residents with ALZ [19]. However, the proposition that TCC may have therapeutic effect as an exercise option for individuals with ALZ requires controlled study.

An electronic search of PubMed revealed no primary clinical research in this area. Continued search of the Internet postings of news media and proceedings of professional conferences yielded information from one pilot study and reports of two demonstration projects. The common focus of this early research is feasibility. An ongoing pilot study being conducted by this author [20] evaluates utility of a program of instruction supplemented with an instructional DVD ('Chi for You, Two, or More ...' Qi Concept Productions, Inc., 2006). Preliminary results reported as conference proceedings found that family caregivers who persisted with Tai Chi-like exercises perceive benefits of relaxation and stress reduction for themselves and behavioral improvement in partners with ALZ. Two additional conference reports, each describe successful implementation of adapted Tai Chi-like exercise programming for individuals with ALZ or dementia. In evaluation of a demonstration project investigating exercise in an adult day care setting, Noyes et al. [21] found that some individuals in middle stages of ALZ disease were able to participate in volunteer-led group classes which included Tai Chi-like exercises while others needed one-on-one exercise guidance provided by exercise aides. Another demonstration project [22] successfully piloted in long-term care settings used a train-the-trainer approach, providing instructional resources to develop facility staff as leaders of Tai Chi-like exercises. The program of exercise, titled CAREx [23], an acronym for

Table 1. Practice-based programming goals and strategies for adapting TCC for individuals with PD and ALZ by stage of disease

	PD	ALZ
Early stage	No accommodation may be needed – integrate into community classes as much as possible.	Rather than traditional forms practice, repeat movement patterns or simple combinations as choreographed practice. Integrate dynamic Qigong movement patterns into practice. Use trained caregivers or volunteers as exercise partners or leaders for small group and one-on-one practice. Evaluate level of participation rather than perfection of form. Establish a quiet controlled environment. Daily or BID practice may be as long as 30–45 min or as little as 5–10 min. Instruct primarily through visual cues and verbal reference to familiar functional tasks such as 'reaching up into the cupboard for picking fruit'. Soft Tai Chi wands or foam balls (10–12 inch in diameter) may be used to add variety to play and to allow participants to more easily follow movement patterns as well as to assist in learning connectedness, position sense.
Middle stages	Welcoming, slower-paced classes. Use arm swinging (repeated trunk rotation) to unlock trunk and pelvis. Emphasize mental aspect and body control, balance training and backwards walking, body and trunk turning coordination. Use instruction aids e.g. soft Tai Chi wand and simplified partner practice. Use verbal or tactile cues to help with any occurrences of 'freezing'. Allow time for socializing.	Programming content and structure is generally the same as early stage. Familiarity with exercises is based on procedural motor memory. Consider seated and sit-to-stand programming. Lead by demonstration. Individuals with late middle stage ALZ who may choose to join in intermittently or passively can benefit through calming and socialization effects.
Late stage	Seated or standing with guarding or ready support. Emphasize breathing regulation and calming aspects. Provide for socialization.	Programming is generally the same as late middle stages. Social, behavioral, and meditative benefits may still be experienced even if physical participation is no longer evident.

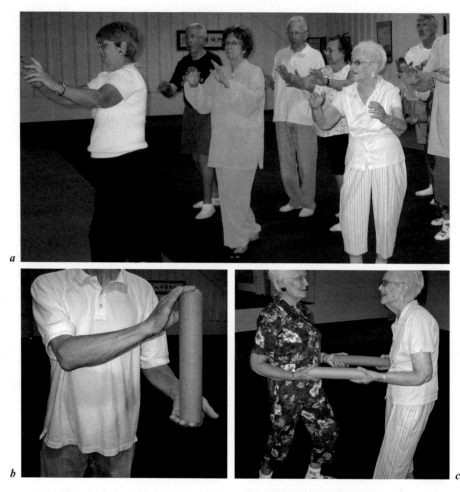

Fig. 1. ***a*** Taiji Buddies class, Buffalo, N.Y., perform repetitions of 'prayer wheel'. Class led by P.J. Klein, Ed.D., P.T., includes, but is not limited to, individuals with PD and their exercise support partners (taiji buddies). Goals of the class are to engage in regular practice of mind/body exercise. Participation cost is covered under health and wellness benefits of at least two major health insurers. Class description, sample routine demonstrations and commentary by class participants is available in DVD format at www.chitime.info. ***b*** Example of 'taiji wand'. Class member holding the wand joined the class as part of his rehabilitation 10 days after deep brain stimulation surgery. Since that time, he and his wife have been regularly attending members of the class. ***c*** Example of partner practice by a mother/daughter pair. Mother on the right is 94 years old. Both have been participating in the class for 3 years considering it to be a heath-promoting social activity.

'calming and relaxing exercises', consists of easy-to-follow, repeated movement patterns and postures which flow one into another adapted from TCC and Qigong.

TCC and ALZ: Clinical Impressions

The few published accounts of demonstration projects [20–22] reviewed in this chapter suggest using easy-to-follow, Tai Chi-like exercise rather than traditional TCC practice for individuals with ALZ. Several additional clinical impressions arise from this work. These include the following. Potential benefits appear to include behavioral, functional and cognitive effect. The slow pace and functional origin of movement patterns characteristic of TCC practice may make Tai Chi-like exercises easier for individuals with ALZ to perform as compared to other exercise options. The general health benefits of physical activity may be gained if sufficient minutes of exercise occur daily. Upper extremity patterns may preserve shoulder flexibility required for self care. Repeated trunk rotations which occur as a part of many of the movement patterns such as 'gazing-at-the-moon' may have an internal massage effect similar to what is experienced in walking which can benefit individuals with limited walking ability. All three models use caregivers (formal and informal) as exercise leaders. This strategy has been found to be successful in home health care [24]. Future research might investigate evidence of benefit to caregiver leaders as well as the individuals with ALZ.

Table 1 lists practice-based recommendations for adaptation of Tai Chi-like exercise for individuals with ALZ. These include cuing procedural movement patterns by recalling familiar functional tasks such as 'reaching up into the cupboard for the TCC exercise' known as 'picking fruit'. Inclusion of reaching exercises aids in maintenance of flexibility and trunk control. Soft Tai Chi wands made of foam tubes can be used to assist in learning connectedness and position sense or as an aid in simply following the movement pattern. Finally, emphasis is on participation and enjoying the calming experience rather than perfection of form. Integrate Qigong movement patterns into practice. In the later stage of the disease or on given days the individual with ALZ may not physically participate, rather the engagement may be social and psychological in the form of observation.

Conclusions

Research evidence investigating effect of TCC practice for individuals with PD is limited in number and weak in design. Suggested outcomes for future study include falls prevention, mobility maintenance, motor control and volitional influence of tremor, breathing regulation, and promotion of well being. Research into utility of TCC as an exercise option for individuals with ALZ is in its very early stages. However, using Tai Chi-like exercises rather than traditional TCC practice appears to be most appropriate for these clinical populations. Hopefully, continued interest in assessing feasibility of adapting TCC and Tai Chi-like programming for these two clinical populations will result in a more informative research base to guide future practice.

Acknowledgment

The author wishes to thank the Taiji Buddies, Buffalo, NY, for their assistance in the reflective genesis of clinical impressions described in this chapter.

References

1   National Institute of Neurological Disorders and Stroke. NINDS Parkinson's Disease: Hope through Research. [cited 2007 Jul 16]. Available at http://www.ninds.nih.gov/disorders/parkinsons_disease/detail_parkinsons_disease.htm.
2   Cummings Jl: Treatment of Alzheimer's disease. Clin Cornerstone 2001;3:27–39.
3   Kristjanson LJ, Aoun SM, Oldham L: Palliative care and support for people with neurodegenerative conditions and their carers. Int J Palliat Nurs 2006;12:368–377.
4   Chodzko-Zajko W, Jahnke R: National Expert Meeting on Qi Gong and Tai Chi Consensus Report. 2006 [cited 2007 Jul 16]. Available at http://www.agingblueprint.org/PDFs/ Consensus Doc.pdf.
5   Brandabur M, Marjama-Lyons J: Complimentary Therapies and Parkinson's. 2000 [cited 2007 July 16]. Available at http://www.parkinson.org/NETCOMMUNITY/Page.aspx?&pid+46l&srcid = 198.
6   Douglas B: Parkinson's Disease & Tai Chi Therapy. 2005 [cited 2007 Jul 16]. Available at http://www.worldtaichiday.org/LIBRARYArticles/LIBRARYTaiChiPARKINSONS.html.
7   Parkinson I, Milligan C: The benefits of T'ai Chi. J Dement Care 2004;12:10–11. [cited 2007 Jul 16] available at http://www.parkinsons.ca/managing.html#taich.
8   Marjama-Lyons J, Smith L, Nelson J, Holiday G, Seracino D: [abstract P190]. Movement Disorders 2002;17:S70.
9   Li F, Harmer P, Fisher KJ, Junheng X, Fitzgerald K, Vongjaturapat N: Tai Chi-based exercise for older adults with Parkinson's disease: a pilot-program evaluation. J Aging Phys Act 2007;15: 139–151.
10 Klein PJ, Rivers LC: Taiji for individuals with Parkinson's and their support partners: Program Evaluation. J Neuro Phy Ther 2006;30:22–27.
11 Kluding P: Multi-dimensional exercise for people with Parkinson's disease: a case report. Physiother Theory Pract 2006;22:153–162.
12 Venglar M: Case Report: Tai Chi and Parkinsonism. Physiother Res Int 2005;10:116–121.
13 Reuters health: Tai chi may help people with Parkinson's disease. 2002 [cited 2007 Jul 16] available at http://www.dotaichi.com/Articles/TaiChiMayHelpParkinson.htm viewed.
14 O'Sullivan SB: Parkinson's disease; in O'Sullivan SB, Schmitz TJ (eds), Physical Rehabilitation, ed 4. FA Davis, 2001, pp 747–782.
15 Gatts SK, Woollacott MH: Neural mechanisms underlying balance improvement with short term Tai Chi training. Aging Clin Exp Res 2006;18:7–19.

16   Knott M, Voss D: Proprioceptive Neuromuscular Facilitation: Patterns and Techniques. New York: Harper & Row, 1968.

17   Lautenschlager NT, Almeida OP: Physical activity and cognition in old age. Curr Opin Psychiatry 2006;19:190–193.

18   Alexopoulos GS, Jeste DV, Chung H, Carpenter D, Ross, R, Docherty JP: The expert consensus guidelines series. Treatment of dementia and its behavioral disturbances. Introduction: methods, commentary, and summary. Postgrad Med 2005;Spec no: 6–22.

19   Rolland Y, Pillard F, Klapouszczak A, Reynish E, Thomas D, Andrieu S, Rivière D, Vellas B: Exercise program for nursing home residents with Alzheimer's disease: a 1-year randomized, controlled trial. J Am Geriatr Soc 2007;55:158–165.

20   Klein PJ: Chi for You: health-promoting exercise. Festival of International Conferences on Caregiving, Disability, Aging and Technology (FICCDAT) Toronto, ONT Jun 16–19, 2007.

21   Noyes L, Wong R, Bellamy-Brown M: Implementing A Group Exercise Program In An Adult Daycare Center For Individuals With Alzheimer's Disease. [Poster] Annual Conference of the American Physical Therapy Association, Jun 30–Jul 3 2004; Chicago, IL, [cited 2007 Jul 16] Available from http://www.apta.org/am/abstracts/pt2004/abstractsPt2004.cfm?pubNo = PO-SI-45-TH.

22   Klein PJ: CAREx: Calming and Relaxing Mind/body Exercises. Festival of International Conferences on Caregiving, Disability, Aging and Technology (FICCDAT) Toronto, ONT Jun 16–19, 2007.

23   Klein PJ, Svensson L, Adams W: CAREx Exercise Leader Training Kit. Qi Concept Publications, Inc: Elma, NY, 2007 Available at www.chitime.info.

24   Logsden RG, McCurry SM, Teri L: A home health care approach to exercise for persons with Alzheimer's disease. Care Manag J 2005;6:90–97.

Penelope J. Klein
Professor of Physical Therapy
D'Youville College, 320 Porter Ave.
Buffalo, NY 14201 (USA)
Tel. +1 716 829 7835, Fax +1 716 829 8137, E-Mail kleinpj@dyc.edu

Hong Y (ed): Tai Chi Chuan. State of the Art in International Research.
Med Sport Sci. Basel, Karger, 2008, vol 52, pp 182–194

· ·

Tai Chi Training for Patients with Coronary Heart Disease

Ching Lan[a], *Ssu-Yuan Chen*[a], *May-Kuen Wong*[b], *Jin-Shin Lai*[a]

[a]Department of Physical Medicine and Rehabilitation, National Taiwan University Hospital and College of Medicine, National Taiwan University, and [b]Department of Physical Medicine and Rehabilitation, Chang-Gung Memorial Hospital and Department of Physical Therapy, Post-Graduate Institute of Rehabilitation Science, Chang-Gung University, Taipei, Taiwan, ROC

Abstract

Coronary heart disease (CHD) is the leading cause of death in the developed countries and many developing countries. Exercise training is the cornerstone of cardiac rehabilitation program for patients with CHD, and exercise intensities in the 50–70% heart rate reserve have been shown to improve functional capacity. However, recent studies found exercise with lower intensity also displayed benefits to CHD patients, and increased the acceptance of exercise program, particularly unfit and elderly patients. Tai Chi Chuan (TC) is a traditional conditioning exercise in the Chinese community, and recently it has become more popular in the Western societies. The exercise intensity of TC is low to moderate, depending on the training style, posture and duration. Participants can choose to perform a complete set of TC or selected movements according to their needs. Previous research substantiates that TC enhances aerobic capacity, muscular strength, endothelial function and psychological well-being. In addition, TC reduces some cardiovascular risk factors, such as hypertension and dyslipidemia. Recent studies have also proved that TC is safe and effective for patients with myocardial infarction, coronary bypass surgery and heart failure. Therefore, TC may be prescribed as an alternative exercise program for selected patients with cardiovascular diseases. In conclusion, TC has potential benefits for patients with CHD, and is appropriate for implementation in the community.

Cardiovascular disease (CVD) is the leading cause of morbidity and mortality in developed countries. In developing countries, the prevalence of CVD also increases rapidly owing to fast economic growth and lifestyles change. Coronary heart disease (CHD), the major category of CVD, is manifest as angina pectoris, acute myocardial infarction (AMI) and sudden cardiac death. From 1985 to 1992, the CHD mortality rate in men aged 35–44 years increased from 4.3/100,000 to 11.4/100,000 in South Korea, and from 4.1/100,000 to 7.8/100,000 in Taiwan [1]. Since 1992, the mortality related to CHD slightly decreased in Taiwan due to improved cardiac care, but the hospitalization rates for CHD significantly increased from 1996 to 2001 [2]. In China, a recent study reported that the rates of CHD mortality in Beijing increased by 50% in men and 27% in women from 1984 to 1999, and 77% of this increase might be attributed to substantial rises in cholesterol levels [3].

Exercise training is the core component of cardiac rehabilitation for patients with CHD. The prescribed exercise intensity should be above a certain level to induce an effective training effect, yet below the metabolic load evokes abnormal clinical signs and symptoms [4]. Moderate-intensity exercises have been shown to improve functional capacity in cardiac patients, and it also provides suitable safety during unsupervised training. However, lower intensity exercise increases the acceptance of training, particularly for unfit and elderly patients. From the standpoint of exercise promotion, some oriental conditioning exercises deserve more attention because they are less intense, easily accessible, low cost and therefore suitable for implementation in the community.

Tai Chi Chuan (TC) is a Chinese mind-body exercise. Recent studies have shown that TC is beneficial to aerobic capacity [5–7], muscular strength [8, 9], and some cardiovascular risk factors [10–14]. Further, TC appears to be safe and effective for patients with AMI, coronary artery bypass grafting (CABG) surgery and congestive heart failure (CHF). Therefore, TC may be prescribed as an alternative exercise program for patients with CHD. This chapter reviews the effect of TC on cardiovascular health based on the existing literature, and introduces the potential application of TC in patients with CHD.

Tai Chi Training

Training Characteristics
TC is a branch of ancient martial arts that has been popular in the Chinese society for several hundred years. TC is well known for its slow and graceful movements, and the training doctrine is deeply rooted in Taoism. The goal of Taoism is to achieve longevity through mind and body training. During the practice, deep diaphragmatic breathing is integrated to complex body motions to achieve a harmonious balance between body and mind. There are many TC styles, among them Chen TC is the oldest, and Yang TC is the most popular [15]. TC is performed in a semi-squat posture, and the exercise intensity can be easily adjusted by controlling the postural height (fig. 1). The characteristics of

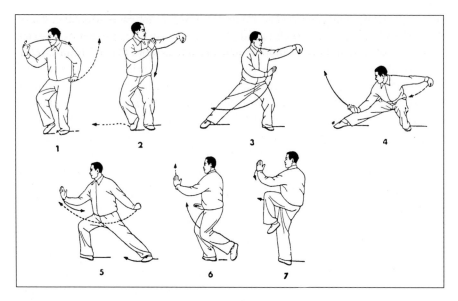

Fig. 1. An example of a typical TC form (push down and stand on one leg). The sequential motions are performed in a semi-squat posture. Reproduced with permission from China Sports [58].

TC are: mind concentration with breathing control; whole body exercise in semi-squat posture; continuous, curved and spiral body movements [15]. Each training session of classical Yang TC includes 20 min of warm-up, 24 min of TC practice, and 10 min of cool-down. Warm-up exercises usually include 10 movements including range of motion exercises, stretching, and balance exercises with 10–20 repetitions.

Exercise Intensity

The exercise intensity of TC depends on the training style, posture and duration. Variation in training approaches results in substantial differences in exercise intensity. Participants may practice selected movements instead of a complete set of TC to improve balance or flexibility. However, if the training goal is to increase aerobic capacity or muscular strength, a complete set of classical TC is recommended.

In a recent study, we used a K4 telemetry system to measure heart rate (HR) responses and oxygen uptake ($\dot{V}O_2$) while performing classical Yang TC in middle-aged men [16]. The HR during TC practice was 58% of the HR reserve, and the $\dot{V}O_2$ during practice was 55% of the peak oxygen uptake

($\dot{V}O_{2peak}$). Additionally, we found the HR during TC practice was 50–58% of HR reserve in males and females aged 25–80 years, which indicated its exercise intensity was similar across different ages in each gender [17]. TC is an aerobic exercise with moderate exercise intensity, and it fulfills the recommendations of the American College of Sports Medicine regarding exercise to develop and maintain cardiorespiratory fitness [18]. Other studies reported the energy cost during TC practice was between 4.1 and 4.6 metabolic equivalents in young participants [19]. For a simplified form of TC, the estimated exercise intensity may decrease to 2.9 metabolic equivalents [19]. Because age and functional capacity in CHD patients vary significantly, choosing a TC program with suitable exercise intensity is important to obtain a suitable training effect.

Training Effects of TC

Aerobic Capacity

Aerobic capacity is a strong predictor of cardiac and all-cause mortality in patients with CVD. In a long-term follow-up for 12,169 patients with CHD, Kavanagh et al. [20] compared the risk of death according to their $\dot{V}O_{2peak}$ values during graded exercise testing. $\dot{V}O_{2peak}$ values of 15, 15–22, and >22 ml · kg^{-1} · min^{-1} yielded hazard ratios of 1.00, 0.62, and 0.39 of cardiac death, respectively. Therefore, exercise training is the core component in cardiac rehabilitation because it significantly improves the aerobic capacity and hence reduces mortality.

Long-term TC training may enhance aerobic capacity. In cross-sectional studies, Lan et al. [5] reported that the middle-aged TC group displayed 15.6–26.8% higher $\dot{V}O_{2peak}$ than the control group [21], while elderly TC practitioners showed 18–19% higher $\dot{V}O_{2peak}$ than their sedentary counterparts. Further, long-term TC practitioners displayed slower age-related decline of aerobic capacity than their sedentary counterparts. In a 2-year follow-up study [22], the annual decrease in $\dot{V}O_{2peak}$ was 0.55 in the male TC group and 0.8 ml · kg^{-1} · min^{-1} in the control group. In the females, the TC groups displayed only half of the decline in $\dot{V}O_{2peak}$ compared to the control group (0.3 vs. 0.6 ml · kg^{-1} · min^{-1}). For sedentary individuals, Lan et al. [6] also reported that entering a TC program significantly enhance the aerobic capacity. After 1 year of TC training, elderly men and women might increase $\dot{V}O_{2peak}$ by 16.1 and 21.3%, respectively.

Muscular Strength

Muscular strength and muscular endurance are important to the activities of daily living. However, maximal muscular strength gradually declines after 50 years of age, thus many deconditioned cardiac patients lack the physical strength to perform daily activities. Improvement of muscular strength and endurance enables cardiac patients to perform certain tasks with less physiological stress and aids in maintaining their functional independence. Resistance training appears to decrease cardiac demands during daily activities like carrying or lifting heavy objects [23]. Additionally, resistance training provides an effective method for improving muscular strength, preventing chronic medical conditions, modifying coronary risk factors, and enhancing functional dependence [24].

TC is performed in a semi-squat posture, and combined concentric and eccentric contractions are needed in this posture. The lower the posture, the higher demand will be put on quadriceps, thus significantly improving muscular strength of the lower extremities. Jacobson et al. [25] reported that a 12-week TC program increased muscular strength of knee extensors. We also proved that a 6-month TC program was effective in enhancing isokinetic strength of knee extensors [8]. In that study, the male TC group increased by 15.1–20.0% of the concentric peak torque in knee extensors, while the eccentric peak torque increased by 15.1–23.7%. In the female TC group, the concentric and eccentric peak torque increased by 13.5–24.2 and 18.3–23.8%, respectively. Both TC groups also showed significant increase in the endurance ratio of knee extensors. In a recent study, Wu et al. [9] measured isokinetic muscular strength of knee extensors, and reported that the TC group had higher muscle power than the control group.

Endothelial Function and Microcirculation

Nitric oxide (NO) is an endothelium-dependent vasodilator that has an important role in the vasodilatory response during exercise [26]. Lack of exercise may predispose the coronary arteries to endothelial dysfunction and arthrosclerosis due to low shear stress status. Low shear stress to the vessel wall has been associated with endothelial proliferative status in animal studies [27], and may contribute to the pathogenesis of arthrosclerosis [28, 29]. However, physical conditioning may enhance vascular responsiveness to endothelium-dependent vasodilators, i.e. NO, in skin and skeletal muscle [30].

Regular practice of TC may enhance endothelium-dependent dilation in skin vasculature of older individuals. In a recent study, Wang et al. [31] reported that older TC practitioners displayed a higher skin blood flow and level of plasma NO metabolite than sedentary subjects at rest and after maximal exercise. In addition, TC subjects had higher arterial blood flow and acetylcholine-induced cutaneous perfusion than the sedentary controls.

TC training is also beneficial to microcirculation. By using impedance plethysmography, we measured skin blood flow and vascular conductance in elderly men before and after a maximal exercise [32]. The results showed that the TC group had higher hyperemic arterial inflow, venous capacity, and venous outflow than their sedentary counterparts. The results implied that TC could delay the age-related decline of venous compliance and hyperemic arterial response.

Blood Lipids

Dyslipidemia, or abnormalities in blood lipid and lipoprotein, is a major risk factor of CHD [33]. The prevalence of dyslipidemia increases with age and westernized lifestyle, but regular exercise may ameliorate the trend toward abnormal blood lipid profile. A recent meta-analysis [34] of 31 randomized controlled trials with exercise training reported a significant decrease in total cholesterol, low-density lipoprotein cholesterol (LDL-C), and triglyceride (TG), and an increase in high-density lipoprotein cholesterol (HDL-C). Typically, the changes in blood lipids were small and it was difficult to separate the effects of exercise from confounders. This may be attributed to differences in baseline lipid concentrations, training amount and intensity, changes in body composition, or the adjunctive interventions such as diet or lipid-lowering agents.

In a study reported by Jiang [35], 1 month of TC training induced an increase in HDL-C and HDL-C/TG, but the level of total cholesterol was unchanged. However, Tsai et al. [13] reported that TC might improve whole blood lipid profile in mild hypertensive patients. In that study, 88 patients were randomized into a TC group and a sedentary control group. After 12 weeks of classical Yang TC training, total cholesterol, TG and LDL-C concentration decreased by 15.2, 23.8 and 19.7 mg/dl, respectively. Further, HDL-C increased by 4.7 mg/dl. In a recent randomized controlled study, Thomas et al. [36] reported no significant change in total cholesterol, TG, LDL-C and HDL-C after 12 months of TC training. Nevertheless, these subjects practiced 24-form simplified TC, the exercise intensity and energy expenditure were lower than for the classical 108-form TC, and this might have influenced the training effect. In the future, more studies are needed to elucidate the effect of TC on blood lipids.

Hypertension

Hypertension is the most prevalent form of CVD affecting approximately 1 billion patients worldwide. Hypertension is the major factor contributing to more than one million heart attacks and 500,000 heart attack deaths annually in the United States [37]. Hypertension is also a risk factor for heart failure and peripheral vascular disease. Therefore, lowering BP benefits hypertensive individuals and significantly reduces the morbidity and mortality of CVD. Regular exercise and lifestyle change are the core of current recommendations for prevention and treatment of hypertension. Recent meta-analyses [38, 39] from 54 randomized clinical trials indicated that aerobic exercise might significantly reduce BP, and the reduction appears to be more pronounced in hypertensive subjects (i.e. -7.4 and -5.8 mm Hg for systolic and diastolic BP, respectively) [39].

TC training also shows beneficial effects for patients with high blood pressure. In TC intervention studies, 6- to 12-week training programs significantly decreased systolic and diastolic BP at rest or after exercise [10–14], and hypertensive patients showed the most favorable improvement. The Fraility and Injuries: Cooperative Studies of Intervention Techniques (FICSIT) study in Atlanta reported that TC training could lower systolic BP from 172 to 159 mm Hg after a 12-min walk in older individuals, and the effect of BP reduction is similar between TC and aerobic exercise [40]. The decrease in BP during exercise may lower the rate pressure product, which indicates a decrease in myocardial oxygen demand. In patients after AMI, 8 weeks of TC training program also lowered resting systolic BP by 3 mm Hg and diastolic BP by 2 mm Hg [10]. Different styles of TC appeared to have a similar effect on BP reduction. Tsai et al. [13] applied 108-form Yang TC to mild hypertensive patients, and reported 15.6- and 8.8-mm Hg reductions in systolic and diastolic BP, respectively. Talor-Piliae et al. [11] utilized 24-form simplified TC in hypertensive patients and the effect of BP reduction was similar (18.9 mm Hg in SBP and 8.9 mm Hg in DBP). However, Thomas et al. [36] reported that 12 months of simplified TC training could not induce any significant change in BP. Further studies are needed to substantiate the effect of TC on blood pressure.

HR Variability

Cardiac vagal modulation decreased in various physiological and pathological conditions, such as AMI [41] and heart failure [42]. Cardiac vagal function can be evaluated by spectral HR variability (HRV) analysis, and decreased HRV was found to be associated with poor outcome in cardiac patients [43]. In a recent study, Lu and Kuo [44] reported that TC practitioners displayed higher HRV than their sedentary counterparts, which implied that TC might enhance the vagal modulation and tilt the sympathovagal balance toward decreased sympathetic modulation. In addition, HR, systolic BP, diastolic BP, mean arterial BP and pulse pressure also decreased 30 and 60 min after TC practice. The results showed that TC might increase HRV in healthy individuals and future application to CHD patients may be considered.

Psychological Well-Being

Jin [45] reported that TC training could increase noradrenaline excretion in urine, and decrease salivary cortisol concentration. The results implied that TC could reduce tension, depression, and anxiety. Moreover, the stress reduction effect of TC was similar to walking at a speed of 6 km/h [46]. Brown et al. [47] also reported a 16-week TC program could reduce mood disturbance and improve general mood in women. In the Atlanta subgroup of the clinical trial of FICSIT, Kutner et al. [48] randomized elderly subjects into the Tai Chi, balance training, and exercise education groups. After 4 months of training, the follow-up assessment found only TC subjects reported that their daily activities and their overall life had been affected, but participants of the other two groups did not. The data suggest that when mental as well as physical control is perceived to be enhanced, with a sense of improvement in overall well-being, the motivation to continue exercising also increases.

TC Application in Patients with CHD

Exercise training cardiac rehabilitation for patients with CHD has not been widely implemented in the developing countries. Traditional exercise training highly relied on equipment training, but non-equipment-based rehabilitation programs are the most practical option for developing countries. Furthermore, the type of rehabilitation program should be matched to the needs and resources of each community [49]. Therefore, TC may be used in cardiac rehabilitation programs because it does not need any equipment and can be easily implemented in communities.

Acute Myocardial Infarction
AMI is the most common cause of mortality in patients with CHD. An overview of randomized trials of cardiac rehabilitation with exercise involving 4,554 patients with AMI indicated a 20% reduction of risk for total mortality, a 22% reduction for cardiovascular mortality, and a 25% reduction in the risk for fatal reinfarction [50]. Therefore, patients recovering from AMI are recommended to receive cardiac rehabilitation services. However, most patients find it inconvenient to attend exercise training courses in hospital three times per week, and thereby the participation rate in rehabilitation program is low. TC is easily accessible, and can be practiced in the community as a group exercise. In addition, TC is an exercise with low to moderate intensity, thus patients with AMI may choose TC as an alternative exercise program according to their fitness level. Channer et al. [10] designed an 8-week low-intensity TC program and applied it to patients with AMI. The results displayed that TC was effective in reducing blood pressure, and was safe for patients after AMI.

Coronary Artery Bypass Graft

Patients with CHD who suffer persistent symptoms while receiving medical therapy may be considered for revascularization procedures, such as CABG. CABG for coronary patients aims to increase blood flow to ischemic myocardium beyond an obstructive lesion, and reduce cardiovascular morbidity and mortality. Nevertheless, CABG patients exhibited a 30% decline in $\dot{V}O_{2peak}$ compared to normal subjects owing to the severity of disease, longer deconditioning and postoperative recovery required [7, 21]. The significant decrease in $\dot{V}O_{2peak}$ in patients after CABG may be detrimental to their life adaptation, and hence exercise is important to patients who undergo CABG.

In order to evaluate the training effect of TC, we underwent a 12-month TC program for low-risk patients after CABG. CABG patients participated in a TC program as a maintenance (phase III) rehabilitation program [7]. The TC group practiced classical Yang TC every morning in the community setting, and the control group was advised to walk at least 30 min three times per week. During the performance of TC, the mean HR while performing TC was 48–57% of their HR reserve. After 12 months of training, the TC group showed significant improvement of oxygen uptake at the peak exercise and the ventilatory threshold (VeT). At the peak exercise, the TC group showed a 10.3% increase in $\dot{V}O_{2peak}$ (from 26.2 ± 4.4 to $28.9 \pm 5.0\,ml \cdot kg^{-1} \cdot min^{-1}$) and 11.8% increase in peak work rate (from 135 ± 26 to $151 \pm 28\,W$), while the control group did not show any improvement. Further, the TC group also increased 17.6% in $\dot{V}O_2$ at the VeT, while the control group did not display significant change. The VeT was used initially to assess the endurance with CVD, and it could be used as a noninvasive estimate of lactate threshold [51]. Coyle et al. [52] reported that the $\dot{V}O_{2peak}$ increased less than $\dot{V}O_2$ at the lactate threshold in patients with CHD. It should be noted that even a small increase in $\dot{V}O_2$ at VeT is beneficial to cardiac patients, because it could raise the functional level in activities of daily living.

Congestive Heart Failure

CHF is characterized by the inability of the heart to deliver sufficient oxygenated blood to tissue owing to impairment of cardiac output. CHF can result in abnormalities in skeletal muscle metabolism, neurohormonal responses, vascular and pulmonary function [53]. Exercise training improves functional capacity and symptoms in patients with heart failure and left ventricular systolic dysfunction, but these changes usually occur without changes in left ventricular function [54]. The increase in exercise tolerance may be attributed to increased skeletal muscle oxidative enzymes and improved mitochondrial density [55]. Recent studies proved that low-intensity TC training might be beneficial to patients with CHF. In a noncontrolled study of 5 patients, Fontana et al. [56] reported that Tai Chi Chih could improve quality of life, 6-min walk and symptoms. In another study, Yeh et al. [57] randomized 30 patients into a TC group (with mean ejection fraction of 24 ± 7%) and a control group, and TC participants practiced 5 basic simplified Yang TC movements twice weekly. After 12 weeks of training, patients' functional capacity and quality of life significantly improved. Further, the TC group showed a decrease in serum B-type natriuretic peptide levels, which implied the severity of heart failure might improve after TC training. For patients with CHF, low-intensity exercise such as simplified TC may increase the acceptance. Intermittent training protocol by using selected TC movements is suitable for patients with very low endurance.

Conclusion

There are several reasons to recommend TC as an alternative exercise program for patients with CHD. First, TC does not need special facilities or expensive equipment, and it can be practiced anytime and anywhere. Second, TC is effective in enhancing aerobic capacity, muscular strength and improving cardiovascular risk factors. Third, TC is a low-cost, low-technology exercise, and it can be easily implemented in the community. It is concluded that TC is effective in promoting cardiovascular health, and it can be prescribed as a maintenance exercise program for patients with CHD.

References

1   Sekikawa A, Kuller LH, Ueshima H, et al: Coronary heart disease mortality trends in men in the post World War II birth cohorts aged 35–44 in Japan, South Korea and Taiwan compared with the United States. Int J Epidemiol 1999;28:1044–1049.
2   Cheng Y, Chen KJ, Wang CJ, Chan SH, Chang WC, Chen JH: Secular trends in coronary heart disease mortality, hospitalization rates, and major cardiovascular risk factors in Taiwan, 1971–2001. Int J Cardiol 2005;100:47–52.
3   Critchley J, Liu J, Zhao D, Wei W, Capewell S: Explaining the increase in coronary heart disease mortality in Beijing between 1984 and 1999. Circulation 2004;110:1236–1244.
4   Franklin BA, Gordon S, Timmis GC: Amount of exercise necessary for the patient with coronary artery disease. Am J Cardiol 1992;69:1426–1432.
5   Lan C, Lai JS, Wong MK, Yu ML: Cardiorespiratory function, flexibility, and body composition among geriatric Tai Chi Chuan practitioners. Arch Phys Med Rehabil 1996;77:612–616.
6   Lan C, Lai JS, Chen SY, Wong MK: 12-month Tai Chi training in the elderly: its effect on health fitness. Med Sci Sports Exerc 1998;30:345–351.
7   Lan C, Chen SY, Lai JS, Wong MK: The effect of Tai Chi on cardiorespiratory function in patients with coronary artery bypass surgery. Med Sci Sports Exerc 1999;31:634–638.
8   Lan C, Lai JS, Chen SY, Wong MK: Tai Chi Chuan to improve muscular strength and endurance in elderly individuals: a pilot study. Arch Phys Med Rehabil 2000;81:604–607.
9   Wu G, Zhao F, Zhou X, Wei L: Improvement of isokinetic knee extensor strength and reduction of postural sway in the elderly from long-term Tai Chi exercise. Arch Phys Med Rehabil 2002;83: 1364–1369.

10 Channer KS, Barrow D, Barrow R, Osborne M, Ives G: Changes in haemodynamic parameters following Tai Chi Chuan and aerobic exercise in patients recovering from acute myocardial infarction. Postgrad Med J 1996;72:349–351.

11 Taylor-Piliae RE, Haskell WL, Froelicher ES: Hemodynamic responses to a community-based Tai Chi exercise intervention in ethnic Chinese adults with cardiovascular disease risk factors. Eur J Cardiovasc Nurs 2006;5:165–174.

12 Thornton EW, Sykes KS, Tang WK: Health benefits of Tai Chi exercise: improved balance and blood pressure in middle-aged women. Health Promot Int 2004;19:33–38.

13 Tsai JC, Wang WH, Chan P, et al: The beneficial effects of Tai Chi Chuan on blood pressure and lipid profile and anxiety status in a randomized controlled trial. J Altern Complement Med 2003;9:747–754.

14 Young DR, Appel LJ, Jee S, Miller ER III: The effects of aerobic exercise and T'ai Chi on blood pressure in older people: results of a randomized trial. J Am Geriatr Soc 1999;47:277–284.

15 China Sports: Simplified Taijiquan, ed 2. Beijing: China Publication Center, 1983, pp 1–5.

16 Lan C, Chen SY, Lai JS, Wong MK: Heart rate responses and oxygen consumption during Tai Chi Chuan practice. Am J Chin Med 2001;29:403–410.

17 Lan C, Chen SY, Lai JS: Relative exercise intensity of Tai Chi Chuan is similar in different ages and gender. Am J Chin Med 2004;32:151–160.

18 American College of Sports Medicine Position Stand. The recommended quantity and quality of exercise for developing and maintaining cardiorespiratory and muscular fitness, and flexibility in healthy adults. Med Sci Sports Exerc 1998;30:975–991.

19 Zhuo D, Shephard RJ, Plyley MJ, Davis GM: Cardiorespiratory and metabolic responses during Tai Chi Chuan exercise. Can J Appl Sport Sci 1984;9:7–10.

20 Kavanagh T, Mertens DJ, Hamm LF, et al: Prediction of long-term prognosis in 12 169 men referred for cardiac rehabilitation. Circulation 2002;106:666–671.

21 Lai JS, Wong MK, Lan C, Chong CK, Lien IN: Cardiorespiratory responses of Tai Chi Chuan practitioners and sedentary subjects during cycle ergometry. J Formos Med Assoc 1993;92: 894–899.

22 Lai JS, Lan C, Wong MK, Teng SH: Two-year trends in cardiorespiratory function among older Tai Chi Chuan practitioners and sedentary subjects. J Am Geriatr Soc 1995;43:1222–1227.

23 Hickson RC, Rosenkoetter MA, Brown MM: Strength training effects on aerobic power and short-term endurance. Med Sci Sports Exerc 1980;12:336–339.

24 Pollock ML, Franklin BA, Balady GJ, et al; AHA Science Advisory: Resistance exercise in individuals with and without cardiovascular disease: benefits, rationale, safety, and prescription: An advisory from the Committee on Exercise, Rehabilitation, and Prevention, Council on Clinical Cardiology, American Heart Association; Position paper endorsed by the American College of Sports Medicine. Circulation 2000;101:828–833.

25 Jacobson BH, Chen HC, Cashel C, Guerrero L: The effect of T'ai Chi Chuan training on balance, kinesthetic sense, and strength. Percept Mot Skills 1997;84:27–33.

26 Palmer RM, Ferrige AG, Moncada S: Nitric oxide release accounts for the biological activity of endothelium-derived relaxing factor. Nature 1987;327:524–526.

27 Mondy JS, Lindner V, Miyashiro JK, Berk BC, Dean RH, Geary RL: Platelet-derived growth factor ligand and receptor expression in response to altered blood flow in vivo. Circ Res 1997;81: 320–327.

28 Gimbrone MA Jr: Vascular endothelium: an integrator of pathophysiologic stimuli in atherosclerosis. Am J Cardiol 1995;75:67B–70B.

29 Traub O, Berk BC: Laminar shear stress: mechanisms by which endothelial cells transduce an atheroprotective force. Arterioscler Thromb Vasc Biol 1998;18:677–685.

30 Green DJ, Maiorana A, O'Driscoll G, Taylor R: Effect of exercise training on endothelium-derived nitric oxide function in humans. J Physiol 2004;561:1–25.

31 Wang JS, Lan C, Wong MK: Tai Chi Chuan training to enhance microcirculatory function in healthy elderly men. Arch Phys Med Rehabil 2001;82:1176–1180.

32 Wang JS, Lan C, Chen SY, Wong MK: Tai Chi Chuan training is associated with enhanced endothelium-dependent dilation in skin vasculature of healthy older men. J Am Geriatr Soc 2002;50:1024–1030.

33   Hebert PR, Gaziano JM, Chan KS, Hennekens CH: Cholesterol lowering with statin drugs, risk of stroke, and total mortality. An overview of randomized trials. JAMA 1997;278:313–321.

34   Halbert JA, Silagy CA, Finucane P, Withers RT, Hamdorf PA: Exercise training and blood lipids in hyperlipidemic and normolipidemic adults: a meta-analysis of randomized, controlled trials. Eur J Clin Nutr 1999;53:514–522.

35   Jiang JX: An observation on the effect of Tai Chi Quan on serum HDL-C and other blood lipids. Chin Sports Med 1984;3:99–101.

36   Thomas GN, Hong AW, Tomlinson B, et al: Effects of Tai Chi and resistance training on cardiovascular risk factors in elderly Chinese subjects: a 12-month longitudinal, randomized, controlled intervention study. Clin Endocrinol (Oxf) 2005;63:663–669.

37   National High Blood Pressure Education Program: The Seventh Report of the Joint National Committee on Prevention, Detection, Evaluation, and Treatment of High Blood Pressure (JNC7), 2003.

38   Whelton SP, Chin A, Xin X, He J: Effect of aerobic exercise on blood pressure: a meta-analysis of randomized, controlled trials. Ann Intern Med 2002;136:493–503.

39   Fagard RH: Exercise characteristics and the blood pressure response to dynamic physical training. Med Sci Sports Exerc 2001;33:S484–S492.

40   Wolf SL, Barnhart HX, Kutner NG, McNeely E, Coogler C, Xu T: Reducing frailty and falls in older persons: an investigation of Tai Chi and computerized balance training. Atlanta FICSIT Group. Frailty and Injuries: Cooperative Studies of Intervention Techniques. J Am Geriatr Soc 1996;44:489–497.

41   Bonnemeier H, Hartmann F, Wiegand UK, et al: Heart rate variability in patients with acute myocardial infarction undergoing primary coronary angioplasty. Am J Cardiol 2000;85:815–820.

42   Nolan J, Batin PD, Andrews R, et al: Prospective study of heart rate variability and mortality in chronic heart failure: results of the United Kingdom heart failure evaluation and assessment of risk trial (UK-heart). Circulation 1998;98:1510–1516.

43   La Rovere MT, Bigger JT Jr, Marcus FI, Mortara A, Schwartz PJ: Baroreflex sensitivity and heart-rate variability in prediction of total cardiac mortality after myocardial infarction. ATRAMI (Autonomic Tone and Reflexes After Myocardial Infarction) Investigators. Lancet 1998;351: 478–484.

44   Lu WA, Kuo CD: The effect of Tai Chi Chuan on the autonomic nervous modulation in older persons. Med Sci Sports Exerc 2003;35:1972–1976.

45   Jin P: Changes in heart rate, noradrenaline, cortisol and mood during Tai Chi. J Psychosom Res 1989;33:197–206.

46   Jin P: Efficacy of Tai Chi, brisk walking, meditation, and reading in reducing mental and emotional stress. J Psychosom Res 1992;36:361–370.

47   Brown DR, Wang Y, Ward A, et al: Chronic psychological effects of exercise and exercise plus cognitive strategies. Med Sci Sports Exerc 1995;27:765–775.

48   Kutner NG, Barnhart H, Wolf SL, McNeely E, Xu T: Self-report benefits of Tai Chi practice by older adults. J Gerontol B Psychol Sci Soc Sci 1997;52:242–246.

49   World Health Organization Expert Committee: Rehabilitation after cardiovascular disease, with special emphasis on developing countries. Technique Report Series no. 831. Geneva: World Health Organization, 1993.

50   O'Connor GT, Buring JE, Yusuf S, et al: An overview of randomized trials of rehabilitation with exercise after myocardial infarction. Circulation 1989;80:234–244.

51   Wasserman K, McIlroy MB: Dedecting the threshold of anaerobic metabolism in cardiac patients during exercise. Am J Cardiol 1964;14:844–852.

52   Coyle EF, Martin WH, Ehsani AA, et al: Blood lactate threshold in some well-trained ischemic heart disease patients. J Appl Physiol 1983;54:18–23.

53   Myers JN, Brubaker PH: Chronic heart failure; in American College of Sports Medicine's Exercise Mangement for Persons with Chronic Disease and Disabilities, ed 2. Champaign, IL: Human Kinetics, 2003, pp 64–69.

54   Belardinelli R, Georgiou D, Cianci G, Purcaro A: Randomized, controlled trial of long-term moderate exercise training in chronic heart failure: effects on functional capacity, quality of life, and clinical outcome. Circulation 1999;99:1173–1182.

55 Pina IL, Apstein CS, Balady GJ, et al: Exercise and heart failure: A statement from the American Heart Association Committee on exercise, rehabilitation, and prevention. Circulation 2003;107: 1210–1225.

56 Fontana JA, Colella C, Baas LS, Ghazi F: T'ai Chi Chih as an intervention for heart failure. Nurs Clin North Am 2000;35:1031–1046.

57 Yeh GY, Wood MJ, Lorell BH, et al: Effects of tai chi mind-body movement therapy on functional status and exercise capacity in patients with chronic heart failure: a randomized controlled trial. Am J Med 2004;117:541–548.

58 China Sports: Simplified 'Taijiquan', ed 2. Beijing: China Publications Center, 1983.

Ching Lan, MD
Department of Physical Medicine and Rehabilitation, National Taiwan University Hospital
7, Chung-Shan South Road
Taipei, 10016 Taiwan (ROC)
Tel. +886 2 397 0800, ext. 6760, Fax +886 2 383 2834, E-Mail clan@ntu.edu.tw

Hong Y (ed): Tai Chi Chuan. State of the Art in International Research.
Med Sport Sci. Basel, Karger, 2008, vol 52, pp 195–208

....

T'ai Chi Exercise in Patients with Chronic Heart Failure

Gloria Y. Yeh[a,b]*, Peter M. Wayne*[a]*, Russell S. Phillips*[a,b]

[a]Division for Research and Education in Complementary and Integrative Medical Therapies, Harvard Medical School, and [b]Division of General Medicine and Primary Care, Department of Medicine, Beth Israel Deaconess Medical Center, Boston, Mass., USA

Abstract

Objective: To review the physiological and psychosocial effects of a 12-week T'ai Chi program (TC) in patients with heart failure (HF) as previously reported in a clinical trial. **Methods:** We randomized 30 patients with chronic HF (left ventricular ejection fraction ≤40%) to receive TC plus usual care (n = 15), or usual care alone (wait-list control, n = 15). Outcome measures included quality of life, exercise capacity, B-type natriuretic peptide, catecholamine levels, heart rate variability, and sleep stability. **Results:** The mean age (±SD) of patients was 64 ± 13 years, mean baseline ejection fraction (±SD) was 23 ± 7%, and median New York Heart Association Class was 2 (range 1–4). At 12 weeks, patients who participated in TC showed improved quality of life (mean change −17 ± 11 vs. 8 ± 15, Minnesota Living with HF Questionnaire, p = 0.001), increased exercise capacity (mean change 85 ± 46 vs. −51 ± 58 m, 6-min walk, p = 0.001), and decreased B-type natriuretic peptide (mean change −48 ± 104 vs. 90 ± 333 pg/ml, p = 0.03) compared to the control group. Those who participated in TC also showed improvement in sleep stability (increase in high-frequency coupling +0.05 ± 0.10 vs. −0.06 ± 0.09 proportion of estimated total sleep time, p = 0.04; reduction in low-frequency coupling −0.09 ± 0.09 vs. +0.13 ± 0.13 proportion of estimated total sleep time, p < 0.01), compared to the control group. **Conclusion:** TC may enhance quality of life, exercise capacity, and sleep stability in patients with chronic HF.

Chronic heart failure (HF) is increasing in prevalence as the population ages and is the most common reason for hospital admission among Medicare patients. Approximately 5 million adults in the US are affected, with 550,000 new cases each year [1]. Despite recent therapeutic advances, patients with HF face progressively deteriorating function. Interventions that can improve functional capacity, quality of life, and overall outcome are needed.

Sedentary lifestyles and physical inactivity, particularly in cardiac patients, can lead to deconditioning and exercise intolerance. Historically, it was thought that initiation of exercise in those with HF would exacerbate HF symptoms [2]. On the contrary, recent trials have demonstrated benefits of exercise in these patients, including improved functional capacity, left ventricular hemodynamics, and quality of life, attenuation of neurohormonal activation and ventricular remodeling, and decreased risk of hospitalization and death. These studies, however, have used varied exercises. Current American Heart Association guidelines do not specify a standard exercise prescription for patients with HF; optimal protocols have yet to be defined [2, 3].

T'ai Chi is a mind-body exercise with origins in traditional Chinese martial and healing arts. Reported benefits include increased balance and decreased incidence of falls, increased strength and flexibility, reduced pain and anxiety, improved self-efficacy, and enhanced cardiopulmonary function [4, 5]. Mind-body therapies like T'ai Chi are being increasingly recognized in cardiac rehabilitation programs in the US [6]. Unlike conventional treadmill or bicycle exercise, T'ai Chi incorporates both physical and meditative elements and emphasizes postural alignment, weight shifting, and low-impact, relaxed circular movements. Exercise intensity has been reported to be 2–4 metabolic equivalents, comparable to mild-moderate aerobic exercise [7, 8]. Trials in HF suggest that lower intensity activity may be just as beneficial as exercise of higher intensity [9]. Because of its mild nature, T'ai Chi may be suitable for older or severely deconditioned cardiac patients.

Prior randomized clinical trials of T'ai Chi in patients with HF are lacking. One prospective, noncontrolled study (n = 5) reported improvements in HF-specific quality of life, 6-min walk, and symptoms after a 12-week intervention [6]. Other controlled trials of T'ai Chi have reported improvements in blood pressure in patients after myocardial infarction [10] and increases in peak oxygen uptake ($\dot{V}O_2$) and work rate following coronary bypass surgery [11]. Observational studies of healthy T'ai Chi practitioners (compared to age-matched sedentary controls) have suggested increased peak $\dot{V}O_2$, exercise endurance, cardiac output, and decreased peripheral vascular resistance and adrenergic tone [5].

Our objective was to investigate whether T'ai Chi is beneficial as an adjunctive treatment to usual care for patients with chronic HF in a prospective randomized controlled trial, and to determine the feasibility of a larger trial. Methods and results of this trial have previously been published in the *American Journal of Medicine and Sleep Medicine* and are reviewed here [12, 13].

Methods

Study Design

We enrolled 30 patients from advanced HF clinics at Beth Israel Deaconess Medical Center and Brigham and Women's Hospital in Boston, Mass., USA. Patients were assigned randomly to receive either 12 weeks of T'ai Chi training in addition to usual care, or to usual care alone, without a formal supervised exercise protocol (wait-list control). Usual care included pharmacologic therapy, dietary counseling, and general exercise advice per American Heart Association guidelines [3]. We used permuted block randomization with variable block size to generate treatment assignments. All patients provided written informed consent. Each institution's human subjects review board approved the study protocol.

Study Population

We included patients with chronic HF and left ventricular ejection fraction ≤40% by echocardiography in the past year, and those on a stable medical regimen (no major changes in medications in the past 3 months). We excluded patients with unstable angina, myocardial infarction, or cardiac surgery within the past 3 months, uncontrolled cardiac arrhythmias, major structural valvular disease, current participation in a conventional cardiac rehabilitation program, lower extremity amputation, cognitive dysfunction, and inability to speak English.

Intervention

One-hour group T'ai Chi classes were held twice weekly for 12 weeks (table 1). Guided by similar interventions used in prior trials with elderly patients and those with limited mobility [14], we developed a standard protocol of meditative warm-up exercises followed by five simplified T'ai Chi movements from Master Cheng Man-Ch'ing's Yang-style short form [15]. Warm-up exercises included weight shifting, arm swinging, visualization techniques, and stretches of the neck, shoulders, spine, arms and legs. Exercises focused on releasing tension in the physical body, incorporating mindfulness and imagery into movement, increasing awareness of breathing and promoting overall relaxation of body and mind. Patients were allowed to progress at their own comfort and pace. Classes were supervised by a physician. Patients were encouraged to practice at home three times per week and received a 35-min instructional video that outlined movements presented in class.

Main Outcome Measures

All measures were obtained at baseline and 12 weeks. The quality of life assessment, 6-min walk, and neurohormone levels were also obtained at 6 weeks in the event that data at 12 weeks were unavailable.

Table 1. Outline and overview of the T'ai Chi intervention

Week	Activities	Approximate duration, min
1	**Introductory session: overview of program**	
	1. T'ai Chi principles, philosophies	15
	2. Demonstration of T'ai Chi form	10
	3. Expectations of participants	10
	4. Description of class format	5
	5. Participation in warm-up exercises	30
2–5	**Warm-up exercises (repeated during all sessions)**	
	1. Standing:	
	a. 'Drumming the body'	6
	b. 'Swinging to connect kidney and lungs'	3
	c. 'Washing the body with qi'	3
	d. Standing meditation and breathing	3
	2. Sitting:	
	a. Neck/shoulder stretches	6
	b. Arm/leg stretches	3
	c. Sitting meditation and breathing	6
	Total warm-up time	30
	T'ai Chi movements	
	1. 'Raising the Power'	5–10
	2. 'Withdraw and Push'	5 per side
	(Warm-up and movements 1–2)	
	3. 'Grasp Sparrows Tail'	5 per side
	4. 'Brush Knee Twist Step'	5 per side
10–12	(Warm-up and movements 1–4)	
	5. 'Wave Hands Like Clouds'	5–10

Reprinted with permission from Yeh et al. [12].

Quality of Life

Quality of life was measured using Minnesota Living with HF Questionnaire, a standardized instrument assessing physical, psychological, and socioeconomic dimensions of illness. Scores range from 0–105, with a lower score denoting a more favorable functional status [16]. Prior studies have reported a score of seven indicates some degree of impaired quality of life and an improvement of five points represents a clinically meaningful change [2].

Exercise Capacity

Patients performed a standardized 6-min walk test. This test correlates with peak $\dot{V}O_2$, and has been used to assess functional capacity and predict survival in HF drug trials [17]. In addition, patients performed a symptom-limited bicycle exercise test to determine peak $\dot{V}O_2$. Testing was performed by a blinded assessor. Breath-by-breath respiratory gas analysis was performed using a Sensormedic metabolic cart (Yorba Linda, Calif., USA). Peak values were averaged from the final 20 s of the test. Peak $\dot{V}O_2$ has a strong linear correlation with cardiac output and skeletal muscle blood flow and is used to predict when patients with chronic HF should undergo cardiac transplantation [18].

Secondary Outcome Measures

Neurohormones
B-type natriuretic peptide (BNP) was analyzed on whole blood collected in EDTA using the Biosite Triage BNP Test (San Diego, Calif., USA) fluorescence immunoassay. Levels of this cardiac biomarker correlate positively with degree of left ventricular dysfunction. Serum levels >100 pg/ml support a diagnosis of symptomatic HF [19].

Catecholamine samples were drawn on ice in heparinized tubes after 20-min rest with intravenous catheter in place. After centrifugation, plasma was separated and stored at −70°C. Analyses for norepinephrine, epinephrine, and dopamine were performed using high-performance liquid chromatography/electrochemical detector.

Continuous Ambulatory Electrocardiographic Recording and Heart Rate Variability
Patients underwent 24-hour ambulatory electrocardiographic (ECG) monitoring to assess cardiac arrhythmias and heart rate variability (HRV). Recordings were performed using Marquette Electronics (Milwaukee, Wisc., USA) series 8500 Holter monitor, digitized at 128 Hz. Annotations were manually verified and edited by a blinded technician.

For standard HRV, 27 of 30 patients provided two complete sets of ECG data. Of these, 9 were excluded from analysis: 2 patients had a nonsinus rhythm and 7 patients were paced. In addition to 24-hour analysis, HRV statistics were separately calculated for sleep and waking activity. Sleep was defined as the 6 night-time hours of lowest heart rate (providing estimated total sleep time, ETST). Waking activity was defined as the 6 daytime hours of highest heart rate. Time and frequency domain HRV statistics were calculated, including average of all normal sinus-to-normal sinus NN intervals (AVNN), standard deviation SD of all NN intervals (SDNN), square root of mean of squares of differences between adjacent NN intervals (rMSSD), percentage of differences between adjacent NN intervals greater than 10–50 ms (pNN10–50), LF (0.04–0.15 Hz), HF (0.15–0.4 Hz), and LF/HF ratio [20, 21]. Complete HRV methods are detailed elsewhere [13].

Spectrographic Analysis of Sleep Stability
We retrospectively analyzed 24-hour ECG data from the 18 subjects who provided 2 complete sets of data, who were not paced, and who were in sinus rhythm. Using a previously described technique, individual sleep spectrograms describing cardiopulmonary coupling were generated that demonstrate periods of stability and instability [22]. A preponderance of power in the low frequency band is associated with instability and periodic sleep behaviors, while excess power in the high frequency band is associated with physiologic respiratory sinus arrhythmia and stable/deep sleep. Low- and high-frequency coupling regimes have weak correlations with standard sleep staging but more closely follow cyclic alternating pattern (CAP) scoring. Low-frequency coupling is associated with CAP and high-frequency coupling with non-CAP. Details of the sleep spectrogram technique are reported elsewhere [13].

Statistical Analysis

All statistical analyses were performed on an intention-to-treat basis. Baseline characteristics of the study patients were compared using t tests for continuous variables and Fisher's exact test for nominal variables. Two-sample Wilcoxon rank-sum tests adjusted for baseline scores were used to compare the distribution of changes after 12 weeks between the intervention and control groups. In addition, we compared within-group pre-post HRV statistics using Wilcoxon rank-sum tests. Metabolic stress test and Holter data for 3 patients in the control group were unavailable at 12 weeks. One patient was too debilitated to perform the tests, one refused, and one was only available for phone follow-up. For the latter patient, we were also unable to gather 6-min walk, BNP, and catecholamine measurements at 12 weeks. For these missing data, the last value was carried forward for analysis.

Results

Subject Characteristics

The mean age of study patients was 64 ± 13 years. There was an equal gender distribution. The mean left ventricular ejection fraction was $23 \pm 7\%$ (table 2). Most patients were on consensus-guided medical therapy. There were no statistically significant differences between the groups with regard to demographics, clinical factors, and rates of cardiovascular-related disease. Rates of other comorbid conditions were also similar, with the exception of arthritis, which was more prevalent in the intervention group (60 vs. 7%, $p < 0.01$). Anxiety/depression was relatively common (~40% both groups). There were no significant differences between the overall study population and the subset of patients examined in HRV and sleep analyses (n = 18). At baseline, 77% of patients reported some regular physical activity at home, such as walking (range 5–65 min, 1–7 times per week).

Quality of Life, Exercise Capacity, and Neurohormones

Those who participated in T'ai Chi (n = 15) showed significantly improved quality of life score (-17 ± 11 vs. 8 ± 15, $p < 0.01$), 6-min walk distance (85 ± 46 m vs. -51 ± 58 m, $p < 0.01$) and serum BNP levels (-48 ± 104 vs. 90 ± 333, $p = 0.03$) compared to the control group (n = 15). Changes in peak oxygen uptake did not reach statistical significance, although the intervention group showed almost 1 ml/kg/min improvement, while the control group showed 0.7 ml/kg/min deterioration (table 3). There were no significant trends seen in resting catecholamine levels.

Table 2. Baseline characteristics of the study sample

	T'ai Chi (n = 15)	Control (n = 15)	p value
Demographic factors			
Age, years	66 ± 12	61 ± 14	0.67
Men	10 (67)	9 (60)	0.71
Race:			0.28
Black	7 (47)	4 (27)	
White	8 (53)	9 (60)	
Asian	0	2 (13)	
Clinical factors			
Baseline ejection fraction, %	24 ± 7	22 ± 8	0.43
New York Heart Association class score	2.2 ± 1.0	2.2 ± 0.6	0.19
Class I	4 (27)	1 (6.6)	
Class II	6 (40)	9 (60)	
Class III	3 (20)	5 (33)	
Class IV	2 (13)	0	
Medications:			
Angiotensin-converting enzyme inhibitor	13 (87)	14 (93)	0.54
β-Blocker	14 (93)	13 (87)	0.54
Loop diuretic	13 (87)	15 (100)	0.48
Digoxin	11 (73)	8 (53)	0.45
Spironolactone	4 (27)	4 (27)	1.00
Cholesterol-lowering agent	5 (33)	6 (40)	0.70
HF etiology			0.79
Idiopathic dilated	9 (60)	8 (53)	
Ischemic	4 (27)	4 (27)	
Alcohol-related	1 (7)	1 (7)	
Hypertensive	0	1 (7)	
Peripartum	1 (7)	0	
Adriamycin-induced	0	1 (7)	
Cardiovascular-related comorbidities			
Coronary artery disease	4 (27)	7 (47)	0.45
Implanted cardiac device[1]	6 (40)	4 (27)	0.70
Arrhythmia	10 (67)	6 (40)	0.27
Valvular heart disease	7 (47)	3 (20)	0.25
Hypertension	11 (73)	9 (60)	0.70
Diabetes	3 (20)	5 (33)	0.68

Reprinted with permission from Yeh et al. [12]. Values in parentheses indicate percentages. Values for age, baseline ejection fraction and New York Heart association class score are expressed as mean ± SD.

[1] Automatic implanted cardiac defibrillator and/or pacemaker.

Table 3. Comparison of the effects of T'ai Chi versus control on mean change in outcome (±SD) during the 12-week trial

Outcome measure	T'ai Chi (n = 15)		Control (n = 15)[1]		Between group difference in change (95% CI)	p value
	Baseline	12-week	Baseline	12-week		
Minnesota Living with Heart Failure[2]	43 ± 21	26 ± 23	44 ± 20	52 ± 25	−25 (−36, −14)	0.001
6-min walk, m	327 ± 106	412 ± 116	340 ± 117	289 ± 165	+135 (+85, +185)	0.001
Peak oxygen uptake, ml/kg/min	10.5 ± 3	11.4 ± 3	11.1 ± 6	10.4 ± 6	+1.6 (+0.2, +3)	0.08
Serum BNP[2], pg/ml	329 ± 377	281 ± 365	285 ± 340	375 ± 429	−138 (−257, −19)	0.03
Plasma norepinephrine, ng/ml	1.3 ± 0.7	1.9 ± 2.3	1.2 ± 0.8	1.4 ± 0.7	+0.35 (−0.84, +1.54)	0.77

Reprinted with permission from Yeh et al. [12].

[1] Imputation methods (last value carried forward) were used for missing 12-week data, affecting 1 patient in the control group for Minnesota Living with Heart Failure score and serum BNP, and 3 patients in the control group for peak oxygen uptake.

[2] For these measures a lower value is better. Thus, a negative between-group difference in change suggests improvement in Minnesota Living with Heart Failure score and B-type natriuretic peptide, while a positive value suggests improvement in 6-min walk.

Continuous ECG Recordings

Standard HRV

Twenty-four-hour Holter monitoring revealed no clinically important intraindividual differences in incidence of arrhythmia at baseline and 12 weeks.

There were no statistically significant changes seen in the 24-hour HRV analyses. However, the T'ai Chi group showed trends toward increased pNN values during sleep that were not seen in the control group. There was a marginally significant increase in pNN30 ($+10.2 \pm 12.1$, $p = 0.049$) in the T'ai Chi group with pNN10, pNN20 and pNN40 approaching significance at $p = 0.079$, 0.060 and 0.054, respectively.

Sleep Spectrograms

After 12 weeks, in the T'ai Chi group, statistically significant improvements were seen in sleep stability, with increases in high-frequency coupling (stable sleep state: $+0.05 \pm 0.10$ vs. -0.06 ± 0.09 proportion of ETST, $p = 0.04$) and reductions in low-frequency coupling (unstable sleep state: -0.09 ± 0.09 vs. $+0.13 \pm 0.13$ proportion of ETST, $p < 0.01$), as compared to the control group. Figure 1 illustrates the effect of T'ai Chi on the ECG-derived sleep spectrogram of a representative patient, with an increase in high-frequency coupling following 12 weeks of T'ai Chi.

Safety/Compliance

No adverse events occurred during class sessions. During the study period, 1 patient in the T'ai Chi group and 4 patients in the control group were hospitalized for HF exacerbation; no deaths occurred. We did not detect any significant changes in mean blood pressure (119/72 mm Hg before vs. 117/72 after) or heart rate (75 beats per min before vs. 73 after) immediately before and after a T'ai Chi session.

Patients in the T'ai Chi group attended 83% of classes, and 93% reported home practice (mean duration 85.5 min per week). All patients rated the classes highly (4 on a 0–4 visual analog scale for enjoyment), and 14 of 15 patients planned to continue T'ai Chi after the study.

Discussion

There is a growing interest in the application of T'ai Chi for patients with HF. According to a recent report on National Institutes of Health research perspectives,

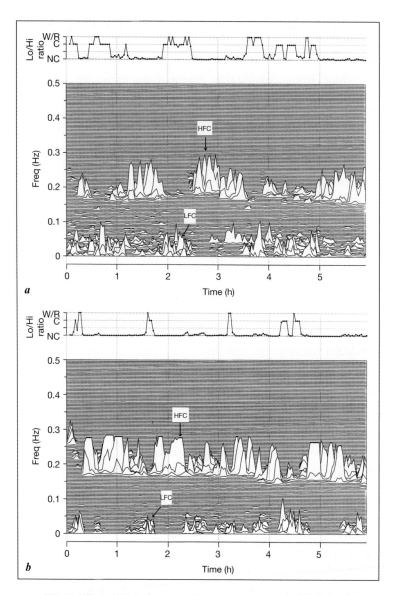

Fig. 1. Effect of T'ai Chi on the sleep spectrogram. ***a*** ECG-derived sleep spectrogram at baseline for a single patient. Note high-frequency (stable sleep state) and low-frequency (unstable sleep state) cardiopulmonary coupling and spontaneous switching between states. ***b*** Increase in high-frequency coupling following the T'ai Chi exposure. This change is evident across the night, and is thus distinctly different from the type of information that can be obtained from standard sleep scoring approaches. Specifically, slow-wave (delta) sleep is an increasingly small percentage of total sleep time in older adults and would thus be less useful in this assessment. C = Cyclic alternating pattern; LFC = low-frequency coupling;

application of complementary therapies to cardiovascular diseases is a funding priority, and T'ai Chi is listed among areas of interest [23]. This chapter presents previously published data from the only randomized controlled trial to date on T'ai Chi exercise in patients with HF.

In summary, we found that a 12-week T'ai Chi program can enhance the quality of life and functional capacity in patients with chronic HF who are already managed with standard medical therapy. Patients who participated in T'ai Chi improved their 6-min walk distances and quality of life scores compared to patients who did not practice T'ai Chi. We also observed a decrease in BNP levels, suggesting an improvement in cardiac filling pressures after T'ai Chi. With traditional HRV measures, there was a trend towards increased short-term HRV during sleep in the T'ai Chi group, suggesting an improvement in cardiac vagal modulation.

In patients with comparable HF severity, similar changes in exercise tolerance have been shown with conventional exercise. Trials using step aerobics, treadmill, bicycle, arm or rowing ergometer have reported increases of 10–20% in 6-min walk distance and increases of 12–31% in peak $\dot{V}O_2$ [24]. With T'ai Chi, we report a comparable increase of ~25% in 6-min walk distance. Results of quality of life measures in conventional exercise trials have been mixed [24, 25], while we report significant improvements. Similar to our findings, conventional exercise trials have failed to show consistent changes in resting norepinephrine and epinephrine [24, 26].

In the retrospective sleep analysis, we found that a 12-week T'ai Chi program can improve sleep stability. An increase in stable sleep may be a robust marker of overall improved sleep quality. For patients with HF, unstable sleep may cause excessive hemodynamic stress through respiratory and nonrespiratory mechanisms, and may be associated with ventricular arrhythmias [27]. In contrast, stable sleep is associated with stable respiration and hemodynamics and may protect from triggered arrhythmias. Improvements in sleep stability may have potentially important restorative effects on chronic HF pathophysiology.

Sleep stability has not previously been described with T'ai Chi, although one prior trial reported improvements in sleep quality, latency, and duration after 24 weeks of T'ai Chi compared to conventional low-impact exercise [28]. Changes in sleep quality have also been demonstrated with other meditative practices, such as mindfulness-based stress reduction and yoga [29, 30].

NC = noncyclic alternating pattern; HFC = high-frequency coupling; W/R = wake or REM sleep, all derived from a single channel of ECG [5]. As polysomnographic data were not available, the sleep period was defined as the 6 night-time hours of the 24-hour period with the lowest mean heart rate. Reprinted with permission from Yeh et al. [13].

T'ai Chi appears to be a safe alternative to conventional exercise. Adverse events in the T'ai Chi literature are lacking. In conventional exercise trials, cases of worsened HF, arrhythmias, and hypotension have been reported, and minor musculoskeletal injuries are common [2]. In contrast, T'ai Chi encourages patients to move fluidly with less strain and may be beneficial for patients with musculoskeletal conditions [5].

While we report encouraging preliminary results, we recognize important study limitations. First, our sample was small and likely underpowered to detect differences in certain measures, e.g. peak $\dot{V}O_2$ and standard HRV. With a wait-list control, patients were not blinded to treatment assignment, and we were unable to control for social interaction. Any social effect on mood or perceived quality of life, however, would be unlikely to account for the magnitude of change we observed in exercise capacity. For the retrospective sleep analysis, polysomnographic data were not available to correlate our results.

In many ways, T'ai Chi appears to be an optimal exercise for patients with HF. T'ai Chi's gentle, low-impact, nonstrenuous movements may be suitable for persons with a wide range of functional capacities, including the elderly and more severely deconditioned, e.g. NYHA Class IV patients. Emphases on efficient breathing and stress reduction also address important cardiorespiratory processes. Further, T'ai Chi can be practiced in any environment, and requires no equipment, possibly offering a cost advantage. Despite this favorable profile and promising preliminary evidence, the exact mechanisms of T'ai Chi are not well understood.

Ongoing investigations at Harvard Medical School and Beth Israel Deaconess Medical Center in Boston continue to explore the role of T'ai Chi exercise in the care of patients with HF. Currently, a larger randomized controlled trial is underway that includes an attention-matched comparison, controlling for group social effect. In addition to exercise capacity and quality-of-life, an expanded list of outcomes includes left ventricular hemodynamics, serum biomarkers of cardiac and immune function, mood, and exercise self-efficacy. Other investigations are comparing T'ai Chi with conventional aerobic exercise, and qualitative analyses are exploring patient experiences, expectations, and belief systems. Further studies might also define the population most likely to benefit from meditative exercise and investigate whether benefits can be sustained or increased. Clearly, T'ai Chi is a rich, complex, multimodal intervention. The challenge will be to design research studies that can appropriately study such an intervention and provide us meaningful insights regarding meditative exercise and its potential application in a clinical setting.

References

1   American Heart Association: Heart disease and stroke statistics- 2003 update. Dallas, Texas: American Heart Association. www.americanheart.org, 2002.

2   Pina IL, Apstein CS, Balady GJ, et al: Exercise and heart failure: a statement from the American Heart Association Committee on exercise, rehabilitation, and prevention. Circulation 2003;107: 1210–1225.

3   Hunt SA, Abraham WT, Chin MH, et al: ACC/AHA 2005 Guideline Update for the Diagnosis and Management of Chronic Heart Failure in the Adult: a report of the American College of Cardiology/American Heart Association Task Force on Practice Guidelines (Writing Committee to Update the 2001 Guidelines for the Evaluation and Management of Heart Failure): developed in collaboration with the American College of Chest Physicians and the International Society for Heart and Lung Transplantation: endorsed by the Heart Rhythm Society www.acc.org, 2005.

4   Wu G: Evaluation of the effectiveness of Tai Chi for improving balance and preventing falls in the older population–a review. J Am Geriatr Soc 2002;50:746–754.

5   Wang C, Collet JP, Lau J: The effect of Tai Chi on health outcomes in patients with chronic conditions: a systematic review. Arch Intern Med 2004;164:493–501.

6   Fontana JA, Colella C: Tai Chi chih as an intervention for heart failure. Nurs Clin North Am 2000;35:1031–1461.

7   Fontana JA, Colella C: The energy costs of a modified Tai Chi exercise. Nurs Res 2000;49:145.

8   Schneider D, Leung R: Metabolic and cardiorespiratory responses to the performance of Wing Chun and Tai Chi Chuan excrcise. Int J Sports Med 1991;12:319–323.

9   Meyer K, Samek L, Schwaibold M: Physical response to different modes of interval exercise in patients with chronic heart failure- application to exercise training. Eur Heart J 1996;17:1040–1047.

10   Channer KS, Barrow D, Barrow R: Changes in haemodynamic parameters following Tai Chi Chuan and aerobic exercise in patients recovering from acute myocardial infarction. Postgrad Med 1996;72:349–351.

11   Lan C, Chen SY: The effect of Tai Chi on cardiorespiratory function in patients with coronary artery bypass surgery. Med Sci Sports Exerc 1999;31:634–638.

12   Yeh GY, Wood MJ, Lorell BH, Stevenson LW, Goldberger AL, Wayne PM, Eisenberg DM, Davis RB, Phillip RS: Effect of Tai Chi mind-body movement therapy on functional status and exercise capacity in patients with chronic heart failure: a randomized controlled trial. Am J Med 2004;117: 541–548.

13   Yeh GY, Mietus JE, Peng CK, Phillips RS, Davis RB, Goldberger AL, Thomas RS: Enhancement of sleep stability with Tai Chi exercise in patients with chronic heart failure: preliminary findings using an ECG-based spectrogram method. Sleep Med 2007, in press.

14   Wolf SL, Coogler C: Exploring the basis for Tai Chi Chuan as a therapeutic exercise approach. Arch Phys Med Rehabil 1997;78:886–892.

15   Cheng MC: T'ai Chi Ch'uan: A Simplified Method of Calisthenics for Health and Self Defense. Berkeley, CA: North Atlantic Books, 1981.

16   Rector TS, Cohn JN: Assessment of patient outcome with the Minnesota Living with Heart Failure questionnaire: reliability and validity during a randomized, double-blind, placebo-controlled trial of pimobendan. Am Heart J 1992;124:1017–1025.

17   Zugck C, Kruger C, Durr S: Is the 6 minute walk test a reliable substitute for peak oxygen uptake in patients with dilated cardiomyopathy? Eur Heart J 2000;21:540–549.

18   Myers J, Gullestad L, Vagelos R, et al: Cardiopulmonary exercise testing and prognosis in severe heart failure: 14 mL/kg/min revisited. Am Heart J 2000;131:78–84.

19   Maisel AS, Krishnaswamy P, Nowak RM, et al: Rapid measurement of B-type natriuretic peptide in the emergency diagnosis of heart failure. New Engl J Med 2002;347:161–167.

20   Mietus JE, Peng CK, Henry I, Goldsmith R, Goldberger AL: The pNNx files: re-examining a widely-used heart rate variability measure. Heart 2002;88:378–380.

21   Heart rate variability: standards of measurement, physiological interpretation and clinical use. Task Force of the European Society of Cardiology and the North American Society of Pacing and Electrophysiology. Circulation 1996;93:1043–1065.

22 Thomas RJ, Mietus JE, Peng CK, Goldberger AL: An electrocardiogram-based technique to assess cardiopulmonary coupling during sleep. Sleep 2005;28:1151–1161.

23 Wong SS, Nahin RL: National Center for Complementary and Alternative Medicine perspectives for complementary and alternative medicine research in cardiovascular diseases. Cardiol Rev 2003;11:94–98.

24 Keteyian SJ, Brawner CA, Schairer JR, et al: Effects of training on chronotropic incompetence in patients with heart failure. Am Heart J 1999;138:233–240.

25 Oka RK, DeMarco T, Haskell WL, et al: Impact of a home-based walking and resistance training program on quality of life in patients with heart failure. Am J Cardiol 2000;85:365–369.

26 Kiilavuori K, Naveri H, Leinonen H, Harkonen M: The effects of physical training on hormonal status and exertional hormonal response in patients with chronic congestive heart failure. Eur Heart J 1999;20:456–464.

27 Leung RS, Diep TM, Bowman ME, Lorenzi-Filho G, Bradley TD: Provocation of ventricular ectopy by cheyne-stokes respiration in patients with heart failure. Sleep 2004;27:1337–1343.

28 Li F, Fisher KJ, Harmer P, Irbe D, Tearse RG, Weimer C: Tai Chi and self-rated quality of sleep and daytime sleepiness in older adults: a randomized controlled trial. J Am Geriatr Soc 2004;52:892–900.

29 Carlson Le, Garland SN: Impact of mindfulness-based stress reduction (MBSR) on sleep, mood, stress and fatigue symptoms in cancer outpatients. Int J Behav Med 2005;12:278–285.

30 Cohen L, Warnecke C, Fouladi RT, Rodríguez MA, Chaoul-Reich A: Psychological adjustment and sleep quality in a randomized trial of the effects of a Tibetan yoga intervention in patients with lymphoma. Cancer 2004;100:2253–2260.

Gloria Y. Yeh, MD, MPH
Harvard Medical School Osher Research Center
401 Park Drive, Suite 22A
Boston, MA 02215 (USA)
Tel. +1 617 384 8550, Fax +1 617 384 8555, E-Mail gyeh@hms.harvard.edu

Hong Y (ed): Tai Chi Chuan. State of the Art in International Research.
Med Sport Sci. Basel, Karger, 2008, vol 52, pp 209–217

....

Tai Chi Chuan for Breast Cancer Survivors

Karen M. Mustian, Oxana G. Palesh, Stephanie A. Flecksteiner

Behavioral Medicine Unit, Department of Radiation Oncology, James P. Wilmot
Cancer Center, University of Rochester School of Medicine and Dentistry, Rochester,
N.Y., USA

Abstract

Background/Aims: Treatment for breast cancer produces side effects that diminish
functional capacity and quality of life (QOL) among survivors. Tai Chi Chuan (TCC) is a
moderate form of exercise that may improve functional capacity and QOL in these individuals. Women who completed treatment for breast cancer were randomized to receive TCC or
psychosocial support therapy for 12 weeks (60 min; three times weekly). **Results:** The TCC
group demonstrated significant improvements in functional capacity, including aerobic
capacity, muscular strength, and flexibility, as well as QOL; the psychosocial support therapy
group showed significant improvements only in flexibility, with declines in aerobic capacity,
muscular strength, and QOL. **Conclusions:** The TCC group exhibited significant improvements in functional capacity and QOL. These data suggest that TCC may enhance functional
capacity and QOL among breast cancer survivors.

According to the American Cancer Society, survival rates for patients with
breast cancer have been increasing dramatically; the 5-plus-year survival of
women diagnosed with localized disease is 97% [1]. Unfortunately, however,
these women experience side effects from their cancer treatments that persist
for years. Exercise may be a safe method for improving quality of life (QOL)
among breast cancer survivors [2–6].

Although few studies have examined physical exercise patterns during and
after treatments for cancer, it appears that patients decrease the amount of physical exercise in which they engage after diagnosis and during treatment. Studies
found that exercise increases following treatment but it does not return to the
prediagnosis level [2, 3, 5, 6]. Several groups have studied the impact of exercise interventions on functional capacity among breast cancer survivors [2, 3,
6]. These exercise studies utilized traditional modes of exercise (e.g. walking,

cycling), and their long-term adherence rates were typically quite low [2, 3, 6]. Novel, alternative modes of physical exercise may better address the unique needs of breast cancer survivors and facilitate increased exercise (re)adoption and adherence.

Tai Chi Chuan (TCC), a practice that is rapidly gaining popularity in the United States [7–11], is a form of exercise that may benefit breast cancer survivors. TCC has shown positive effects on QOL and components of health-related fitness, such as cardiorespiratory function, strength, and flexibility in individuals without cancer [8, 10, 12, 13]. The purpose of this study was to conduct an initial test of the efficacy and appropriateness of a TCC intervention by comparing the benefits of a 12-week TCC program against a 12-week psychosocial support therapy (PST) program (exercise control group) on functional capacity (e.g. aerobic capacity, muscular strength, flexibility) and QOL in breast cancer survivors.

Methods

Subjects

Women who completed treatments for breast cancer were recruited for this study. To participate in the study, individuals were required to meet the following inclusion criteria: (1) be female; (2) have a diagnosis of primary breast cancer stage 0–IIIb; (3) be between 1 week and 30 months after treatment; (4) have no drainage tubes or catheters; (5) engage in moderate to vigorous physical activity no more than once a week; (6) have a physician's clearance for fitness testing and exercise; (7) have no physical limitations prohibiting exercise, and (8) have no clinical diagnoses of mental disorders, as defined by the use of psychotropic drugs and self-report.

Design and Procedures

Participants were randomly assigned to a 12-week TCC exercise group or PST typical care control group. Each group met three times a week for 60 min. The PST sessions were facilitated by a trained counselor and an Exercise Psychology graduate student and conducted in an open-ended format that placed strong emphasis on teaching behavioral coping strategies, peer support, and group cohesion. Participants in the PST group were instructed not to begin any physical exercise programs or change their normal daily physical activity in any way for the duration of the study.

The TCC group was led by an American College of Sports Medicine Certified Health and Fitness Instructor with extensive training in Yang-style TCC. Participants performed 10 min of warm-up stretching and basic Chi Kung (stationary TCC fundamentals). The participants then performed TCC for approximately 40 min and learned a 15-move short-form sequence of Yang-style TCC. The 15 moves used in the current study intervention consisted of the first 15 moves of the traditional 104-move Yang-style long form. During the final 10 min of each session, participants were instructed in regulatory breathing, imagery, and meditation in order to enhance their TCC skills and provide an exercise cool-down. Participants in the TCC group were instructed not to begin any other physical exercise programs and not to change their normal daily physical activity during the course of the study [12, 13].

Measures

All of the testing protocols adhered to procedures and guidelines set forth by the American College of Sports Medicine (ACSM). All tests were conducted by ACSM-certified personnel. Functional capacity was assessed by evaluating three domains of health-related physical fitness: aerobic capacity, muscular strength, and flexibility. Aerobic capacity was estimated using a 6-min walk test protocol that has been used extensively in clinical exercise trials [14, 15]. Muscular strength was evaluated using a handgrip dynamometer to assess the maximal voluntary grip strength [15]. Although not a direct measure, handgrip dynamometry is correlated with overall body strength [15]. Flexibility was assessed using goniometer measurements of shoulder flexion, extension, abduction, and adduction [15]. QOL was measured using the Functional Assessment of Chronic Illness Therapy-Fatigue survey, a 28-item scale developed specifically for use in cancer clinical trials [16]. Adherence and compliance were monitored using attendance rosters, facilitators' process notes and participants' home journals.

Results

Participants

Twenty-one women completed the study. Eleven TCC participants had a 72% exercise attendance rate with 100% compliance and ten PST group participants had a 67% PST attendance rate with 100% compliance during the sessions attended. The reasons expressed by participants for discontinuing included not liking their group assignment, work-family issues, joining a fitness center, severe side effects from treatment (e.g. cognitive deficits), and scheduling conflicts.

Participants ranged in age from 33 to 78 years old (mean = 52 years; SD = 9). The average height and weight were 164 cm (SD = 6) and 70 kg (SD = 12.8), respectively. The average body mass index was 26.3 (SD = 4.9), and average body fat percentage was 41.5 (SD = 5.7) as assessed by bioelectrical impedance at baseline. Almost half the women were married, (48%). Most were Caucasian (90%), had at least some college education (90%), were employed outside the home (65%), and had household incomes above USD 40,000 (62%). All of the participants were diagnosed with stage 0–IIIb breast cancer and had received surgical treatment (61% lumpectomy, 33% mastectomy, 6% bilateral mastectomy). The majority also had received at least one additional treatment modality: chemotherapy (84%), radiation therapy (61%), or hormonal therapy (56%). Statistical comparisons, using independent t tests,

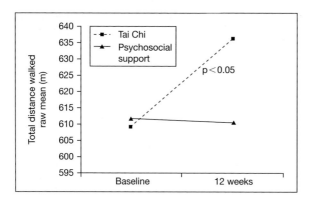

Fig. 1. Comparison between TCC and PST in mean change from baseline to week 12 in total distance walked.

showed no differences (p > 0.05) between participants in the two randomized groups on these baseline characteristics. An additional thorough review of participant records yielded no noticeable differences among the participants who withdrew from the study and participants who did not withdraw.

Functional Capacity

Aerobic Capacity

A 2 × 2 (condition by time) repeated-measures ANOVA, with total distance walked (meters) during the 6-min walk test as the dependent variable, revealed a time by condition interaction effect that approached conventional levels for statistical significance ($F_{1, 19}$ = 3.507; p = 0.077), suggesting a trend. Follow-up repeated-measures ANOVAs, with the data split based on intervention assignment, showed significant improvements in distance walked across the 12-week period among the TCC participants ($F_{1, 10}$ = 5.733; p = 0.038; mean change = 26.93; SD = 37.30; ES = 0.46), with decreases in distance walked among the PST group participants (p > 0.05; mean change = −1.35; SD = 31.23; ES = −0.02; fig. 1).

Baseline and postintervention means and confidence intervals for all functional capacity domains and QOL are provided in table 1.

Muscular Strength

A 2 × 2 (condition by time) repeated-measures ANOVA, with handgrip strength (kilograms) as the dependent variable, revealed a significant time by condition interaction ($F_{1, 19}$ = 9.144; p = 0.007), as well as a significant time

---

Table 1. Means and 95% confidence intervals at baseline and 12 weeks for aerobic capacity, strength, flexibility, and QOL

	Mean at baseline				Mean at 12 weeks			
	TCC (n = 11)		PST (n = 10)		TCC (n = 11)		PST (n = 10)	
	mean	CI	mean	CI	mean	CI	mean	CI
Aerobic capacity (total distance walked), m	609.1	564.0–654.3	611.6	555.1–668.3	636.12	602.7–669.5	610.3	556.0–664.5
Strength, kg	24.5	21.7–28.7	27.5	22.7–32.3	29.6	27.4–32.0	26.7	22.6–30.8
Flexibility, degrees								
Flexion	128.1	116.3–140.1	125.8	116.9–134.7	144.3	135.1–153.6	132.1	122.3–141.8
Extension	43.3	35.7–50.9	44.4	36.3–52.4	68.9	60.2–77.6	51.4	39.7–63.0
Abduction	158.4	144.9–172.1	154.2	140.5–167.8	174.2	165.9–182.8	165.0	152.4–177.5
Horizontal adduction	26.8	21.3–32.5	23.7	19.9–27.4	38.9	32.6–45.2	26.3	20.4–32.1
Horizontal abduction	97.8	88.9–106.7	96.2	87.6–104.7	103.4	97.1–109.9	98.8	92.3–105.3
QOL	107.5	92.7–122.3	124.7	112.7–136.8	121.7	107.7–135.8	124.3	108.2–140.3

main effect ($F_{1, 19} = 4.256$; p = 0.050). Decomposition of interaction and main effects using follow-up repeated-measures ANOVAs, with the data split based on intervention assignment, indicated significant improvements in handgrip strength across the 12-week period in the TCC group ($F_{1, 10} = 10.034$; p = 0.010; mean change = 4.50; SD = 4.71; ES = 1.08), but not in the PST group which actually showed declines in handgrip strength (p > 0.05; mean change = −0.85; SD = 3.15; ES = −0.13).

Flexibility

A $2 \times 2 \times 5$ (condition by time by outcome) repeated-measures MANOVA, with flexion, extension, abduction, horizontal adduction, and horizontal abduction as the dependent variables, revealed a multivariate time by condition interaction that approached statistical significance ($F_{1, 19} = 2.719$; Wilks' $\lambda = 0.061$), suggesting a trend, as well as a significant multivariate time main effect ($F_{1, 19} = 14.524$; Wilks' $\lambda = 0.000$). Further univariate analyses indicated significant time by condition interactions for extension ($F_{1, 10} = 8.530$; p = 0.009) and horizontal abduction ($F_{1, 10} = 6.832$; p = 0.017), along with significant time main effects for flexion ($F_{1, 10} = 14.831$; p = 0.001), extension ($F_{1, 10} = 26.270$; p = 0.000), abduction ($F_{1, 10} = 32.658$; p = 0.000), horizontal adduction ($F_{1, 10} = 7.527$; p = 0.013), and horizontal abduction ($F_{1, 10} = 16.425$; p = 0.001).

Follow-up repeated-measures ANOVAs, with the data split based on intervention assignment, were also conducted. These measures showed significant improvements across the 12-week period among the TCC participants in flexion ($F_{1, 10} = 12.965$; p = 0.005; mean change = 16.18; SD = 14.91; ES = 1.4), extension ($F_{1, 10} = 34.665$; p = 0.000; mean change = 25.55; SD = 14.39; ES = 2.3), abduction ($F_{1, 10} = 17.185$; p = 0.002; mean change = 15.81; SD = 12.66; ES = 1.2), horizontal adduction ($F_{1, 10} = 6.612$; p = 0.028; mean change = 5.64; SD = 7.27; ES = 9.1), and horizontal abduction ($F_{1, 10} = 18.706$; p = 0.002; mean change = 12.05; SD = 9.24; ES = 1.2). The PST participants showed significant improvement in abduction only ($F_{1, 9} = 18.826$; p = 0.002; mean change = 10.80; SD = 7.87; ES = 0.17), with additional, but not statistically significant, improvements in flexion (p > 0.05; mean change = 6.30; SD = 11.40; ES = 0.64), extension (p > 0.05; mean change = 7.00; SD = 14.69; ES = 0.44), horizontal abduction (p > 0.05; mean change = 2.6; SD = 7.04; ES = 0.17), and horizontal adduction (p > 0.05; mean change = 2.60; SD = 6.39; ES = 0.09).

Quality of Life

A 2×3 (condition by time) repeated-measures ANCOVA, with QOL as the dependent variable and baseline self-esteem as the covariate (due to significant baseline differences between groups), revealed a significant time main effect ($F_{1, 19} = 8.04$; $p = 0.00$). Follow-up repeated measures ANCOVAs, with the data split based on intervention assignment, showed significant improvements in QOL across the 12-week period among the TCC participants ($F_{2, 9} = 4.34$; $p = 0.03$), but not in the PST participants ($F_{2, 8} = 2.66$; $p = 0.14$). Additionally, a one-way ANOVA demonstrated a trend toward significant differences between participants in the TCC and PST conditions on changes in QOL at 12-weeks ($F_{1, 19} = 3.66$; $p = 0.07$), but not at 6 weeks ($F_{1, 19} = 2.07$; $p = 0.17$). Furthermore, the TCC participants reported improvements in QOL at 6 and 12 weeks, while the PST participants reported decreases in QOL at both assessment times.

Discussion

The results of this preliminary investigation suggest that TCC has a positive influence on functional capacity and QOL in women of all ages (33–78) following treatment for breast cancer. The TCC group demonstrated significant improvements at 6 and 12 weeks in aerobic capacity, muscular strength, flexibility, and QOL even in a relatively small sample size of breast cancer survivors. The TCC group had excellent adherence and attendance rates compared to other exercise programs reported in the literature. This suggests that the novel integrative exercise modes have a potential to meet the unique needs of breast cancer survivors and lead to improvements in both physical and emotional well-being domains. More research is warranted given these positive findings in a small group of survivors on the efficacy of TCC for improving other common side effects associated with cancer and its treatments (i.e. depression, anxiety, distress and sleep disturbance).

In contrast, the PST group showed declines at 12 weeks in aerobic capacity and muscular fitness, with significant improvement in abduction and nonsignificant improvements in all other areas of flexibility. The PST group also showed declines in QOL. These findings support and expand previous research showing benefits from exercise following cancer treatments [2–6, 12, 13, 17–26] and suggest that groups that provide social supportive environment for breast cancer survivors might not be as sufficient to address the multiple and complex physical and emotional needs of cancer survivors.

In conclusion, these results provide preliminary evidence that TCC may improve aerobic capacity, muscular strength, and flexibility among cancer survivors as well as QOL. These data suggest that TCC has strong potential as a post-treatment rehabilitative modality for improving functional capacity and facilitating the resumption of an optimal QOL among breast cancer survivors. It is unclear from this pilot intervention which part of the group provided the most benefit (e.g. social interaction, mindfulness components, physical activity). Additional research with a larger sample is needed to further delineate the positive effects of TCC among cancer survivors. Future research should examine the possibility of developing a TCC exercise program for breast cancer patients undergoing treatment given the low intensity of the intervention, the high adherence rates, lack of side effects and positive impact on domains of functional capacity and QOL.

References

1   American Cancer Society: Cancer Facts and Figures. American Cancer Society, 2006.
2   Galvao DA, Newton RU: Review of exercise intervention studies in cancer patients. J Clin Oncol 2005;23:899–909.
3   Knols R, Aaronson N, Uebelhart D, Fransen J, Aufdemkampe G: Physical exercise in cancer patients during and after medical treatment: A systematic review of randomized and controlled clinical trials. J Clin Oncol 2005;23:3830–3842.
4   Mustian KM, Katula JA, Gill DL: Exercise: Complementary therapy for breast cancer rehabilitation. Women Therapy 2002;25:105–118.
5   Mustian KM, Griggs JJ, Morrow GR, et al: Exercise and side effects among 749 patients during and after treatment for cancer: a University of Rochester Cancer Center Community Clinical Oncology Program Study. Support Care Cancer 2006;14:732–741.
6   Stevinson C, Lawlor D, Fox K: Exercise interventions for cancer patients: systematic review of controlled trials. Cancer Causes Control 2004;15:1035–1056.
7   Xu H, Lawson D, Kras A, Ryan D: The use of preventive strategies for bone loss. Am J Chin Med 2005;33:299–306.
8   Wang C, Collet JP, Lau J: The effect of Tai Chi on health outcomes in patients with chronic conditions: a systematic review. Arch Intern Med 2004;164:493–501.
9   Han A, Robinson V, Judd M, Taixiang W, Wells G, Tugwell P: Tai chi for treating rheumatoid arthritis. Cochrane Database Syst Rev 2004;CD004849.
10 Klein PJ, Adams WD: Comprehensive therapeutic benefits of Taiji: a critical review. Am J Phys Med Rehabil 2004;83:735–745.
11 Astin JA, Shapiro SL, Eisenberg DM, Forys KL: Mind-body medicine: state of the science, implications for practice. J Am Board Fam Pract 2003;16:131–147.
12 Mustian KM, Katula JA, Gill DL, Roscoe JA, Lang D, Murphy K: Tai Chi Chuan, health-related quality of life and self-esteem: A randomized trial with breast cancer survivors. Support Care Cancer 2004;12:871–876.
13 Mustian KM, Katula JA, Zhao H: A pilot study to assess the influence of tai chi chuan on functional capacity among breast cancer survivors. J Support Oncol 2006;4:139–145.
14 Solway S, Brooks D, Lacasse Y, Thomas S: A qualitative systematic overview of the measurement properties of functional walk tests used in the cardiorespiratory domain. Chest 2001;119:256–270.
15 American College of Sports Medicine: ACSM's Guidelines for exercise testing and prescription. Baltimore, Lippincott: Williams, & Wilkins, 2006.
16 Cella D, Nowinski CJ: Measuring quality of life in chronic illness: The functional assessment of chronic illness therapy measurement system. Arch Phys Med Rehabil 2002;83:S10–S17.
17 Courneya KS, Friedenreich CM: Physical exercise and quality of life following cancer diagnosis: a literature review. Ann Behav Med 1999;21:171–179.
18 Courneya KS, Friedenreich CM: Framework PEACE: an organizational model for examining physical exercise across the cancer experience. Ann Behav Med 2001;23:263–272.

19   Courneya KS: Exercise interventions during cancer treatment: biopsychosocial outcomes. Exerc Sport Sci Rev 2001;29:60–64.
20   Dimeo F: Radiotherapy-related fatigue and exercise for cancer patients: a review of the literature and suggestions for future research. Front Radiat Ther Oncol 2002;37:49–56.
21   Mock V, Dow KH, Meares CJ, et al: Effects of exercise on fatigue, physical functioning, and emotional distress during radiation therapy for breast cancer. Oncol Nurs Forum 1997;24:991–1000.
22   Pinto BM, Maruyama NC: Exercise in the rehabilitation of breast cancer survivors. Psychooncology 1999;8:191–206.
23   Courneya KS, Friedenreich CM, Sela RA, Quinney HA, Rhodes RE, Handman M: The group psychotherapy and home-based physical exercise (group-hope) trial in cancer survivors: physical fitness and quality of life outcomes. Psychooncology 2003;12:357–374.
24   Mock V, Pickett M, Ropka ME, et al: Fatigue and quality of life outcomes of exercise during cancer treatment. Cancer Pract 2001;9:119–127.
25   Courneya KS, Keats MR, Turner AR: Physical exercise and quality of life in cancer patients following high dose chemotherapy and autologous bone marrow transplantation. Psychooncology 2000;9:127–136.
26   Pinto BM, Trunzo JJ, Reiss P, Shiu S: Exercise participation after diagnosis of breast cancer: Trends and effects on mood and quality of life. Psychooncology 2002;11:1–12.

Karen M. Mustian, PhD
University of Rochester School of Medicine and Dentistry, James P. Wilmot Cancer Center
Department of Radiation Oncology, Behavioral Medicine Unit
601 Elmwood Avenue, Box 704, Rochester, NY 14642 (USA)
Tel. +1 585 273 1796, Fax +1 585 461 5601, E-Mail Karen_Mustian@urmc.rochester.edu

Hong Y (ed): Tai Chi Chuan. State of the Art in International Research.
Med Sport Sci. Basel, Karger, 2008, vol 52, pp 218–229

....

Tai Chi Improves Pain and Functional Status in Adults with Rheumatoid Arthritis: Results of a Pilot Single-Blinded Randomized Controlled Trial

Chenchen Wang

Tufts-New England Medical Center, Boston, Mass., USA

Abstract

Background/Aims: Rheumatoid arthritis (RA) is a serious health problem resulting in significant morbidity and disability. Tai Chi may be beneficial to patients with RA as a result of effects on muscle strength and 'mind-body' interactions. To obtain preliminary data on the effects of Tai Chi on RA, we conducted a pilot randomized controlled trial. Twenty patients with functional class I or II RA were randomly assigned to Tai Chi or attention control in twice-weekly sessions for 12 weeks. The American College of Rheumatology (ACR) 20 response criterion, functional capacity, health-related quality of life and the depression index were assessed. **Results:** At 12 weeks, 5/10 patients (50%) randomized to Tai Chi achieved an ACR 20% response compared with 0/10 (0%) in the control (p = 0.03). Tai Chi had greater improvement in the disability index (p = 0.01), vitality subscale of the Medical Outcome Study Short Form 36 (p = 0.01) and the depression index (p = 0.003). Similar trends to improvement were also observed for disease activity, functional capacity and health-related quality of life. No adverse events were observed and no patients withdrew from the study. **Conclusion:** Tai Chi appears safe and may be beneficial for functional class I or II RA. These promising results warrant further investigation into the potential complementary role of Tai Chi for treatment of RA.

Pain and functional impairment are hallmarks of rheumatoid arthritis (RA), a chronic, progressive, inflammatory systemic disease that causes joint destruction and synovial inflammation, resulting in substantial long-term disability with reduced balance and coordination, aerobic capacity, and muscle strength [1]. Patients with RA have a significantly shorter life expectancy compared with the general population [2]. Treatment and management of RA is a major challenge for both rheumatologists and patients with RA.

Current pharmacological therapy focuses on decreasing inflammatory activity and symptoms, limiting joint destruction and disability and improving health-related quality of life (HRQL), and there is little evidence the therapies reverse loss of function. In addition, the long-term consequence and effectiveness of prolonged therapy with many of these agents is unknown [3].

Since 1975, a growing body of randomized and nonrandomized clinical trials has demonstrated that adequate exercise might play an important role in preventing disability and improving function in patients with RA [4–8]. However, numerous questions remain about the optimal exercise regimen for patients with RA. For example, joint damage has been observed after participating in certain high-impact exercises (such as classic aerobic, strengthening exercises and impact sporting activities) [9–10]. Recently, recommendations from the American College of Rheumatology (ACR) guidelines have changed from high-intensity aerobic exercise to regular physical activity [11].

These promising trends in the potential utility of low-impact exercise for patients with RA and the increasing interest in nonpharmacologic therapies for treatment of this chronic disease prompted us to evaluate Tai Chi as a potential complementary therapy for patients with RA. Tai Chi is a traditional Chinese martial art that has been practiced for many centuries [12]. Significant improvements in cardiovascular and respiratory function, balance, strength, flexibility and arthritis symptoms have been reported for a variety of patient populations [13], but the effect of Tai Chi in RA has not been well studied in randomized clinical trials. Although the mechanism of action of Tai Chi is unknown, we hypothesized that Tai Chi may be beneficial to patients with RA as a result of an effect on muscle strength, flexibility, pain, stress and anxiety as well as 'mind-body' interactions [14]. Thus, the goal of this randomized trial was to conduct a preliminary study to evaluate whether 12 weeks of Tai Chi may be a safe and effective complementary therapy for patients with RA.

Methods

Study Design

This pilot study was a prospective, single-blind, randomized controlled clinical trial to evaluate the safety, physical and psychological effects of Tai Chi training for patients suffering from functional class I and II RA [15]. The setting was an urban tertiary care academic hospital in Boston. The study was approved by the Tufts-New England Medical Center (Tufts-NEMC)/Tufts University Human Investigation Review committee and was conducted in the General Clinical Research Center at Tufts-NEMC.

Study Setting and Population

Adults aged 18 and older with functional class I or II RA (ACR criteria [15]) were eligible to participate. The study was conducted between June 2002 and February 2003. Subjects were excluded if they: (1) had prior experience with Tai Chi or other similar types of complementary and alternative medicine such as Qi gong, yoga and acupuncture and/or were unwilling to abstain from participation in Tai Chi (other than that provided for the study) until completion of the study; (2) had cardiovascular or other severe diseases limitations precluding full participation, as determined by the primary care provider; (3) had a mini-mental status score below 24 [16]; (4) were pregnant or breastfeeding; (5) were non-English speaking, and (6) had participated in any other clinical trial within the last 30 days.

There were no eligibility criteria relating to medical therapy for RA. Patients continued routine medications such as NSAIDS, corticosteroids and DMARDs and maintained treatment visits with their primary care physician and rheumatologist throughout the conduct of the study. The investigators recorded any changes made to treatment but did not change or recommend change in medical therapy.

Twenty ambulatory patients with functional class I or II RA were recruited from the outpatient Rheumatology clinic at Tufts and randomly assigned to receive Tai Chi (n = 10) or attention control (n = 10) in twice-weekly 1-hour group sessions for 12 weeks. Randomization assignments were made using computer-generated random numbers, in two groups of 10 and were provided in a sealed, opaque envelope upon agreement to participate. The maximum period between screening and randomization was 3 months.

Tai Chi Intervention

The Tai Chi program was based on classical Yang style [17]. Patients participated in two 60-min Tai Chi sessions conducted each week for 12 weeks. Each session included: (1) 10 min of warm-up and a review of Tai Chi principles; (2) 30 min of Tai Chi exercises; (3) 10 min of breathing technique, and (4) 10 min of relaxation. Subjects were instructed to practice Tai Chi at least 20 min once a day at home. All subjects were encouraged to maintain their usual physical activities, but not to participate in additional strength training other than their Tai Chi exercises.

Stretching and Wellness Education – Control Group

The control group also attended two 60-min sessions per week for 12 weeks. Each session started with 40 min of information about (1) RA as a disease; (2) diet and nutrition; (3) therapies to treat RA, and (4) physical and mental health education (recognizing and dealing with stress and depression, etc.). The final 20 min consisted of stretching exercises involving the upper body, trunk and lower body, each stretch being held for 10–15 s. Subjects were also instructed to practice at least 20 min strength exercises once a day at home. All subjects were encouraged to maintain their usual physical activities, but not to participate in additional strength training other than their class stretching exercises. Throughout the 12-week period, we tracked the number of and reasons for missing sessions in both groups.

Outcome Measures

The primary outcome measure was the proportion of subjects who attained an ACR 20 response criterion at week 12 [18]. ACR 20 is a combined index of response that requires at least 20% improvement in both the tender and swollen joint count, as well as at least 20% improvement in 3 of the 5 following measures: patients' measurement of pain, patient's or physician's global assessment of disease activity, or a physical function measure (the Disability Index of the Health Assessment Questionnaire, HAQ) [19], and serum levels of C-reactive protein (CRP) or erythrocyte sedimentation rate (ESR).

Secondary outcomes included change in the tender and swollen joint scores, the Ritchie Articular Index [20], the Disability Index of the HAQ, 10-cm visual analogue scale (VAS) self-assessment of pain, a 10-cm VAS patient and physician global assessment of disease severity, 10-cm VAS self-assessment of fatigue, ESR, CRP and physical function. The HRQL measure included the Medical Outcome Study Short Form 36 (SF-36) [21], and the EuroQol (EQ-5D) [22], as well as the Center for Epidemiology Studies Depression (CES-D) index [23].

Functional assessment included grip strength (best of 3; Hand Dynamometer TKK 5401 Grip-D, Takei, Japan), time to complete the 50-foot walk and chair stand (with the tenth repetition, using the best, lowest, score). Medications use, demographic information, current exercise pattern, medical history, daily nutrition questionnaire, and adverse events were also recorded.

The Ritchie Articular Index obtained according to the original description (53 joints in 26 units, graded for tenderness on pressure (0, no pain; 1, patient complains of pain; 2, patient complains of pain and winces; 3, patient complains, winces, and withdraws; maximum score 78), was used to assess the degree of joint tenderness.

The HAQ is self-administered and performance is measured in activities of daily living on 8 subscales, which are averaged to create a disability index ranging from 0 (able without difficulty) to 3 (unable to do). The highest scores in each of the categories are then summed (range 0–24) and divided by the number of categories scored, to give a disability index that ranges from 0 to 3, with higher scores indicating more disability. The HAQ also includes pain in the past week (15-cm visual analog scale that is scored 0–3).

The SF-36 is a widely used, standardized generic instrument with scores that are based on responses to individual questions, which are summarized into 8 scales, each of which measures a health concept. These scales include function domains and aspects of well-being as follows: physical functioning, role-physical, bodily pain, general health, vitality, social function, role-emotional and mental health. Scores for each scale range from 0 to 100, with higher scores reflecting better health status. In addition to the eight scales providing the health profile of the individual, two summary measures are available: physical health measure and mental health measure. These have been standardized to have a mean of 50 and a standard deviation of 10. Higher scores on the scales indicate better HRQL.

The EQ-5D is also a generic measure, which describes health states in terms of five dimensions: mobility (disability), self-care (disability), usual activities (handicap), pain/discomfort (impairment), anxiety/depression (impairment). There is also a visual analogue thermometer rating scale to evaluate the overall perception of health on a 0–100 scale. The EQ-5D has been shown to possess high reliability and validity.

The CES-D has been demonstrated to have acceptable levels of reliability and validity. It includes 20-item Likert-type scale used to assess depressive symptoms. The CES-D has high internal consistency (r = 0.85–0.90), test-retest reliability (r = 0.57 for 2–8 weeks), and correlates with clinical ratings of severity of depression. Scores range from 0 to 60, with higher scores indicating greater dysphoria.

All outcome measures were administered at baseline and 12 weeks and 3-month telephone follow-up. Physical examination (a full joint assessment for pain and swelling according to the ACR guidelines) and functional capacities were blindly assessed by the study rheumatologist and a physiologist.

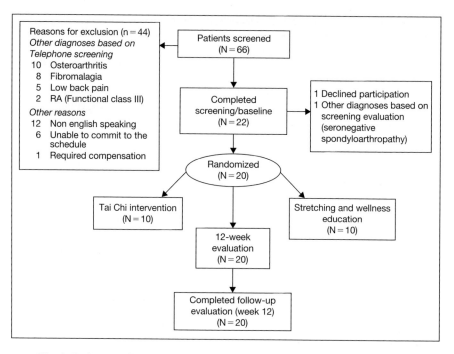

Fig. 1. Patient enrollment.

Statistical Considerations

This pilot study was intended to provide preliminary descriptive data on the potential effect of Tai Chi in patients with RA and therefore the sample size of 20 patients, 10 per group, was empiric. Between groups, continuous variables were compared using the Wilcoxon rank-sum test and binary variables were compared using the Fisher exact test. Within groups, we used the Wilcoxon signed-rank statistic to evaluate absolute and relative change in continuous variables. The primary outcome (ACR 20) and clinical examination were compared using an intent-to-treat analysis.

For this preliminary study, we report two-sided p values less than 0.05 as significant without adjustment for multiple testing. All data analysis and testing were performed using package SAS (Cary, N.C., USA) version 8.2.

Results

Patient Population

We screened 66 patients and 22 patients were evaluated at the baseline (fig. 1). Two were ineligible after baseline evaluation – one had seronegative spondyloarthropathy, and one was unable to commit to the study schedule. The

---

Table 1. Baseline demographic and clinical characteristics

	Tai Chi (n = 10)	Control (n = 10)	p value
Age, years	48 ± 10	51 ± 17	0.57
Females	80%	70%	1.00
White race	80%	70%	1.00
BMI	24 ± 6	28 ± 5	0.12
Weight, kg	64 ± 16	82 ± 23	0.08
Regular exercise	70%	90%	0.58
Duration of RA, years	14 ± 6	15 ± 11	0.86
Morning stiffness (>1 h)	50%	50%	1.00
NSAID	90%	60%	0.30
DMARD	60%	90%	0.30
Corticosteroids	30%	20%	1.00
Rheumatoid factor positive	90%	70%	0.58
Hemoglobin, g/dl	13.4 ± 1.6	13.3 ± 1.1	0.78
Albumin, g/dl	3.9 ± 0.3	4.0 ± 0.3	0.56

Values are mean ± SD for continuous variables. BMI = Body mass index; NSAID = nonsteroidal antirheumatic drug; DMARD = disease-modifying antirheumatic drug.

baseline characteristics of the 20 study subjects are presented in table 1. At baseline, the Tai Chi group had significantly worse HAQ scores and CRP, but was similar in other characteristics including pain and ESR (table 1).

Outcomes

At 12 weeks, 5 of 10 (50%) Tai Chi subjects had achieved the ACR 20% response compared with 0 of 10 in the controls (p = 0.03 in the unadjusted model and p = 0.05 in the adjusted model). Among the 5 subjects who achieved ACR 20 in the Tai Chi group, all had improvement in joint tenderness (20–81%), joint swelling (25–80%) and physician's global assessment of disease activity (44–80%). Four subjects had improvement in pain measurements (20–84%), HAQ score (71–100%) and CRP (36–89%). Two Tai Chi subjects had 20% improvement in almost all the variables in the ACR 20 criteria even without considering the 2 variables (HAQ and CRP) that were not balanced between the study groups at baseline, and thus could have biased the statistical analysis.

Table 2 shows mean change in disease activity, disability, and functional capacity; table 3 shows mean change HRQL and depression scores at 12 weeks.

Table 2. Mean changes in disease activity, disability and functional capacity

	Baseline	Week 12	Change from baseline to week 12	p value within group	p value between group
Disease activity, disability					
Tender joints					
Tai Chi	17.0 ± 10.2	11.7 ± 8.1	−5.3 ± 5.9	0.02	0.06
Control	10.7 ± 8.6	11.1 ± 12.3	0.4 ± 6.3	0.95	
Swollen joints					
Tai Chi	13.5 ± 10.6	12.3 ± 10.6	−1.2 ± 5.5	0.44	0.06
Control	6.7 ± 8.0	8.4 ± 9.9	1.7 ± 3.0	0.15	
Ritchie Articular Index					
Tai Chi	0.5 ± 0.4	0.3 ± 0.3	−0.2 ± 0.2	0.04	0.06
Control	0.3 ± 0.3	0.3 ± 0.4	0.04 ± 0.2	0.76	
HAQ Disability Index					
Tai Chi	0.9 ± 0.7*	0.4 ± 0.4	−0.5 ± 0.5	0.02	**0.01**
Control	0.4 ± 0.3*	0.5 ± 0.4	0.1 ± 0.3	0.57	
Pain past week, 0–3 scale[1]					
Tai Chi	1.4 ± 0.8	1.0 ± 0.7	−0.4 ± 0.8	0.13	0.23
Control	0.8 ± 0.5	0.9 ± 0.7	0.2 ± 0.9	0.57	
Pain (current; 10-cm VAS)					
Tai Chi	3.2 ± 2.2	2.3 ± 2.0	−1.0 ± 2.7	0.16	0.12
Control	1.4 ± 1.3	3.0 ± 2.4	1.6 ± 2.8	0.14	
Patient global (10-cm VAS)					
Tai Chi	2.9 ± 2.4	2.4 ± 2.6	−0.5 ± 1.6	0.55	0.59
Control	2.4 ± 1.9	3.2 ± 2.8	0.7 ± 3.1	0.63	
Fatigue (VAS; 10-cm VAS)					
Tai Chi	4.5 ± 2.5	2.9 ± 2.3	−1.5 ± 2.8	0.11	0.31
Control	3.6 ± 3.0	3.1 ± 1.9	−0.5 ± 2.6	0.47	
ESR, mm/h					
Tai Chi	35.3 ± 28.4	35.1 ± 27.6	−0.2 ± 9.1	0.98	0.56
Control	26.8 ± 14.1	30.1 ± 21.3	3.3 ± 13.3	0.55	
CRP, mg/l					
Tai Chi	1.4 ± 0.8*	1.3 ± 1.3	−0.1 ± 1.2	0.65	0.14
Control	0.5 ± 0.4*	0.6 ± 0.5	0.1 ± 0.3	0.15	
Functional Capacity					
Grip strength, kg					
Tai Chi	16.7 ± 9.3	17.7 ± 9.9	9.6 ± 24.9	0.32	0.32
Control	23.3 ± 9.3	22.5 ± 9.0	−3.6 ± 7.3	0.37	
Chair stand time, s					
Tai Chi	26.4 ± 11.7	20.6 ± 6.9	−19.0 ± 11.9	0.01	0.57
Control	25.6 ± 7.3	21.5 ± 7.1	−15.8 ± 12.9	0.04	
50-foot walking time, s					
Tai Chi	10.9 ± 3.2	9.6 ± 3.1	−12.0 ± 8.0	0.01	0.94
Control	11.3 ± 2.5	9.8 ± 1.6	−11.6 ± 12.1	0.03	

Values are given as mean ± SD. * p < 0.05, statistically significant difference at baseline between the Tai Chi and control groups. p values for continuous variables are exact p values from Wilcoxon rank-sum test. p values for categorical variables are from Fisher exact test. All tests are two sided.

[1]The HAQ includes pain in the past week (15-cm VAS with a score range of 0–3).

Table 3. Mean changes in health status and depression index

	Baseline	Week 12	Change from baseline to week 12	p value within group	between group
PCS (0–50)					
Tai Chi	36.4 ± 8.8	42.8 ± 8.2	6.3 ± 9.5	0.11	0.28
Control	41.3 ± 7.1	43.2 ± 9.5	1.9 ± 6.7	0.38	
MCS (0–50)					
Tai Chi	50.5 ± 13.7	56.9 ± 5.4	6.4 ± 12.0	0.16	0.22
Control	54.8 ± 9.2	54.2 ± 9.2	−0.7 ± 8.2	0.69	
SF-36 subscales (0–100)					
Physical functioning					
Tai Chi	57.0 ± 26.7	75.0 ± 16.3	18.0 ± 21.1	0.03	0.37
Control	66.5 ± 16.3	76.3 ± 17.5	9.8 ± 15.2	0.07	
Role-physical					
Tai Chi	47.5 ± 38.1	67.5 ± 39.2	20.0 ± 35.0	0.16	0.11
Control	62.5 ± 41.2	55.0 ± 38.7	−7.5 ± 33.4	0.66	
Bodily Pain					
Tai Chi	50.8 ± 19.4	63.4 ± 16.5	12.6 ± 19.7	0.11	0.75
Control	58.1 ± 12.6	66.1 ± 20.1	8.0 ± 23.9	0.38	
General health					
Tai Chi	55.3 ± 20.1	68.3 ± 18.3	13.0 ± 29.6	0.36	0.57
Control	67.3 ± 17.2	69.0 ± 17.0	1.7 ± 10.9	0.70	
Vitality					
Tai Chi	44.5 ± 23.0	64.0 ± 15.4	19.5 ± 24.2	0.04	**0.01**
Control	60.5 ± 15.4	62.0 ± 16.5	1.5 ± 11.1	0.48	
Social functioning					
Tai Chi	72.5 ± 28.1	85.0 ± 16.5	12.5 ± 23.6	0.16	0.08
Control	88.8 ± 12.4	82.5 ± 17.9	−6.3 ± 13.5	0.25	
Role-emotional					
Tai Chi	70.0 ± 48.3	100.0 ± 0.0	30.0 ± 48.3	0.25	0.14
Control	83.3 ± 32.4	86.7 ± 23.3	3.3 ± 39.9	1.00	
Mental health					
Tai Chi	75.0 ± 24.7	82.0 ± 14.9	7.0 ± 18.6	0.44	1.00
Control	77.6 ± 13.5	79.6 ± 16.2	2.0 ± 6.6	0.29	
EQ-5D Thermometer Rating Scale (0–100)					
Tai Chi	72.4 ± 19.2	78.8 ± 13.8	6.4 ± 24.5	0.31	0.09
Control	84.0 ± 7.9	74.1 ± 17.7	−9.9 ± 18.0	0.13	
CES-D					
Tai Chi	16.6 ± 3.5	14.3 ± 1.9	−2.30 ± 3.2	0.06	**0.003**
Control	13.0 ± 3.6	15.8 ± 4.1	2.80 ± 4.8	0.07	

Values are given as mean ± 1 SD. PCS = Physical component score; MCS = mental component score; CES-D = the Center for Epidemiology Studies Depression.

Overall, the Tai Chi group improved in all 25 secondary outcomes, while the control group improved in only some and never by as great an amount. The Tai Chi group improved significantly more than the control group only on the HAQ disability index (p = 0.01), the vitality subscale of SF-36 (p = 0.01) and the CES-D (p = 0.003). Physical function variables (chair stand and 50-foot walk) improved in both groups (within group comparisons, p < 0.05), but between-group comparisons were not statistically significant. Overall, Tai Chi improved both physical and mental health scores; however, the data suggest a stronger effect on mental than physical components.

Two patients in the Tai Chi group changed their medication during the study period (1 was prescribed DMARD therapy with infliximab and hydroxy-chloroquine and another discontinued infliximab after losing health insurance). Neither subject achieved the ACR 20 response. There were no adverse events associated with Tai Chi or education and stretching training during the 12-week study period. No patients withdrew from the study.

During the 3-month follow-up (telephone interview), 9 patients in the Tai Chi group continued to practice Tai Chi (3 of them joined a Tai Chi class, 6 practiced Tai Chi at home). All 9 patients reported improvement (less joint pain and fatigue) compared to the baseline measurement. One patient did not continue to practice because of flare-up. All 10 patients in the wellness education and stretching exercises group reported that they maintained their healthy diet, and 5 of 10 patients continue to practice stretch exercise at home. Two patients flared up and changed their medication.

Discussion

This preliminary study shows that group Tai Chi is a safe and promising complementary therapy for adults with functional class I or II RA. Specifically, the results demonstrated that Tai Chi seems to be associated with trends toward improvement in disease activity that relates to both symptoms of pain and the cognitive coping process, which in turn is related to physical and psychological disability.

Furthermore, Tai Chi was not only associated with trends to improvement in symptoms of pain, physical function, and disability in RA, but also suggested a strong improvement in depression. However, there are 2 variables (HAQ, CRP) that differed significantly between groups at the baseline measurements, so it appears that analyses of these effects are confounded. Due to the small sample size of this pilot study, we did not attempt to adjust for these baseline differences.

Our results are consistent with two nonrandomized studies of Tai Chi for RA that reported that there was no significant exacerbation of joint symptoms for 10-week Tai Chi [24]. It is also consistent with other Tai Chi studies in which Tai Chi had beneficial effects on tension, anxiety, and depression [13].

The mechanisms by which Tai Chi may influence the disease process of RA are unknown but may include effects on mental health, including stress reduction and relaxation. We hypothesize that the carefully controlled breathing of Tai Chi may result in a rested body, a peaceful mind and progressive relaxation that may break the arthritis 'pain cycle' (pain, stress, depression may all interfere with functional capabilities) [25].

Although this study has demonstrated a substantial difference in the ACR 20 between the two groups, the relationship between exercise and disease activity measures remains unclear. Functional capacity is a major outcome variable of therapeutic effects in RA [26] which is measured by HAQ and functional capacity (grip strength, chair stand, walk time). While patient's self-reported physical function (HAQ) was improved in the Tai Chi group, the objective measures of functional capacity and laboratory measures of disease activity were not significantly different between treatment groups. While this observation is likely explained by the small sample size and the single-blinded nature of the study (patient aware of group assignment), it is possible that patients are feeling better about themselves and believe that they can do more than they actually can. Future studies extending the duration of the Tai Chi intervention and carefully examining psychological adaptations such as self-efficacy and patients sense of control over their disease are warranted. In addition, longer studies should be done to investigate the impact of Tai Chi on joint damage, which we could not assess in this small, 3-month pilot study.

The study was limited by the small sample size; moreover, the Tai Chi group appears to have had more severe RA, as measured by higher HAQ, CRP, and tender joint count at baseline and therefore may have had a greater chance for improvement in the outcome measures. This difference likely occurred by chance as a result of the small sample size for this study, rather than as a problem with the randomization procedures. Thus it may have been easier for the Tai Chi group than for the control group to improve by 20% or more (ACR criteria). The Tai Chi group also weighed less than the controls (table 1), so we cannot exclude that Tai Chi may help joint symptoms in nonobese more than obese individuals.

In spite of these limitations, the rigor of the study design and our promising results warrant further investigation into the potential complementary role of Tai Chi for treatment of RA. The preliminary findings reported here support the idea that Tai Chi is a safe and attractive exercise for improving physical and especially mental health of patients with RA. Therefore, this preliminary work can be used to develop a conceptual framework exploring the mechanisms that influence complex outcomes such as pain, disability, depression and health-related quality of life. Additional studies that measure the mental components of Tai Chi including psychological, neurological, immunological factors would be critical for further understanding the complex pathophysiology of effect of Tai Chi on chronic autoimmune disease such as RA.

Acknowledgements

I am grateful to Drs. Patricia L. Hibberd, Ronenn Roubenoff, Joseph Lau, Robert Kalish, Christopher Schmid, Hocine Tighiouart, Ramel Rones and GCRC nurses for their help with different aspects of the study, and to Barbara Tanenbaum for her expertise in teaching the control group. We gratefully acknowledge the participation of our study subjects; their cooperation, encouragement and enthusiasm was an inspiration to the investigators.

References

1   National Institute of Arthritis and Musculoskeletal and Skin Disease Web site. Available at http://www.niams.nih.gov. Accessed December, 2007.
2   Pincus T, Callahan LF: Reassessment of twelve traditional paradigms concerning the diagnosis, prevalence, morbidity and mortality of rheumatoid arthritis. Scand J Rheumatol Suppl 1989;79: 67–96.
3   Schiff MH, Whelton A: Renal toxicity associated with disease-modifying antirheumatic drugs used for the treatment of rheumatoid arthritis. Semin Arthritis Rheum 2000;30:196–208.
4   Ekblom B, Lovgren O, Alderin M, Fridstrom M, Satterstrom G: Effect of short-term physical training on patients with rheumatoid arthritis I. Scand J Rherumatol 1975;4:80–86.
5   Rall LC, Meydani SN, Kehayias JJ, Dawson-Hughes B, Roubenoff R: The effect of progressive resistance training in rheumatoid arthritis. Increased strength without changes in energy balance or body composition. Arthritis Rheum 1996;39:415–426.
6   Hakkinen A, Sokka T, Kotaniemi A, Hannonen P: A randomized two –year study of the effects of dynamic strength training on muscle strength, disease activity, functional capacity, and bone mineral density in early rheumatoid arthritis. Arthritis Rheum 2001;44:515–522.
7   van den Ende CH, Breedveld FC, le Cessie S, Dijkmans BA, de Mug AW, Hazes JM: Effect of intensive exercise on patients with active rheumatoid arthritis: a randomized clinical trial. Ann Rheum Dis 2000;59:615–621.
8   Stenstrom CH, Minor MA: Evidence for the benefit of aerobic and strengthening exercise in rheumatoid arthritis. Arthritis Rheum 2003;49:428–434.
9   Finickh Al, Iversen M, Liang MH: The exercise prescription in rheumatoid arthritis: primum non nocere. Arthritis Rheum 2003;48:2393–2395.
10 de Jong Z, Munneke M, Zwinderman AH, Kroon HM, Jansen A, Ronday KH, et al: Is a long-term high-intensity exercise program effective and safe in patients with rheumatoid arthritis? Results of a randomized controlled trial. Arthritis Rheum 2003;48:2415–2424.
11 American College of Rheumatology Subcommittee on Rheumatoid Arthritis Guidelines. Guidelines for the management of rheumatoid arthritis: 2002 update. Arthritis Rheum 2002;46: 328–346.
12 Lan C, Lai JS, Chen SY: Tai Chi Chuan: an ancient wisdom on exercise and health promotion. Sports Med 2002;32:217–224.
13 Wang C, Collet J, Lau J: The Effect of Tai Chi on Health Outcomes in Patients with Chronic Conditions: A Systematic Review. Arch Intern Med 2004;164:493–501.
14 Delza S: Tai Chi Chuan: Body and mind in harmony. Rev. ed. Albany, NY: State University of New York Press, 1985.

15 Arnett FC, Edworthy SM, Bloch DA, McShane DJ, Fries JF, Cooper NS, Healey LA, Kaplan SR, Liang MH, Luthra HS, et al: The American Rheumatism Association 1987 revised criteria for the classification of rheumatoid arthritis. Arthritis Rheum 1988;31:315–324.

16 Folstein MF, Folstein SE, McHugh PR: 'Mini-mental state'. A practical method for grading the cognitive state of patients for the clinician. J Psychiatr Res 1975;12:189–198.

17 China Sports: Simplified 'Taijiquan,' ed 2. Beijing: China Publications Center, 1983.

18 Felson DT, Anderson JJ, Boers M, Bombardier C, Furst D, Goldsmith C, et al: American College of Rheumatology. Preliminary definition of improvement in rheumatoid arthritis. Arthritis Rheum 1995;38:727–735.

19 Fries JF, Spitz P, Kraines RG, Holman HR: Measurement of patient outcome in arthritis. Arthritis Rheum 1980;23:137–145.

20 Ritchie DM, Boyle JA, McInnes JM, Jasani MK, Dalakos TG, Grieveson P, et al: Clinical studies with an articular index for the assessment of joint tenderness in patients with rheumatoid arthritis. Q J Med 1968;37:393–406.

21 Ware JE Jr, Sherbourne CD: The MOS 36-item short-form health survey (SF-36). I. Conceptual framework and item selection. Med Care 1992;30:437–483.

22 Hurst NP, Kind P, Ruta DA, Hunter M, Stubbings A: Measuring health-related quality of life in rheumatoid arthritis: validity, responsiveness and reliability of EuroQol (EQ-5D). Br J Rheumatol 1997;36:551–559.

23 Radloff LS: The CES-D scale: A new self-report depression scale for research in the general population. Appl Psychol Meas 1977;1:385–401.

24 Kirsteins AE, Dietz F, Hwang SM: Evaluating the safety and potential use of a weight-bearing exercise, Tai-Chi Chuan, for rheumatoid arthritis patients. Am J Phys Med Rehabil 1991;70: 136–141.

25 Yocum DE, Castro WL, Cornett M: Exercise, education, and behavioral modification as alternative therapy for pain and stress in rheumatic disease. Rheum Dis Clin North Am 2000;26:145–159.

26 Hazes JM, van den Ende CH: How vigorously should we exercise our rheumatoid arthritis patients? Ann Rheum Dis 1996;55:861–862.

Chenchen Wang, MD, MSc
Assistant Professor of Medicine
Division of Rheumatology
Tufts-New England Medical Center
Box 406, Boston, MA 02111 (USA)
Tel. +1 617 636 3251, Fax +1 617 636 1542, E-Mail cwang2@tufts-nemc.org

Hong Y (ed): Tai Chi Chuan. State of the Art in International Research.
Med Sport Sci. Basel, Karger, 2008, vol 52, pp 230–238

··················

Effects of Tai Chi Exercise on Patients with Type 2 Diabetes

Jing Hao Wang

Faculty of Sports Science, South China Normal University, Guangzhou, China

---

Abstract

This study investigated the effects of Tai Chi exercise on the levels of blood glucose, insulin and insulin receptors of patients with type 2 diabetes. Twelve subjects aged 58–75 years old (66.5 ± 8.5 years) with type 2 diabetes participated in the study. They were trained with the protocol of Tai Chi exercise for 8 weeks. Blood glucose, serum insulin, and insulin receptor activity were measured before and after the 8-week intervention and immediately after a single bout exercise of Tai Chi after the protocol. The results showed that by 8 weeks of Tai Chi exercise, the blood glucose decreased ($p < 0.05$), while high- and low-affinity insulin receptor numbers (r_1, r_2) and low-affinity insulin receptor binding capacity (R_2) increased. Serum insulin increased ($p < 0.05$) but was still within the normal range. After the single bout Tai Chi exercise, blood glucose, high- and low-affinity insulin receptor numbers (r_1, r_2), and their binding capacity (R_1, R_2) increased ($p < 0.05$), while serum insulin did not change. The 8-week Tai Chi intervention therefore showed benefits on health status of patients with type 2 diabetes.

Diabetes mellitus (DM) is a metabolic disease affecting the regulation of insulin and glucose, thereby causing a disruption in the normal control of counter-regulatory hormones and macronutrients and resulting in blood glucose accumulation. Metabolic deregulation leads to the production of noxious substances that have a particular propensity for damaging vascular and nervous structures [1]. Physiological changes with aging as observed are responsible for chronic degenerative diseases which are correlated with a concomitant increase in DM and its associated complications, particularly cardiovascular disease and diabetic nephropathy. The mortality of patients with diabetes is, in most instances, related to these complications [2]. In 2000, the World Health Organization (WHO) estimated that 177 million people were suffering from DM. This shows a 31% increase over 5 years, which is up from 135 million in 1995, and an astonishing 490% increase over the 1985 estimate of 30 million. The WHO projects 350 million people will suffer from diabetes by 2030, and that DM may account for 9% of the total global causes of death. Furthermore, with a projected prevalence increase of 134% within the next 25 years among individuals over the age of 65 years, it will require costly medical procedures and may impose an even larger financial burden on the social system in the USA [3]. Therefore, the primary prevention of DM would avoid the extremely high costs of treatment for the end stage of the disease [4].

It is reported that subjects with type 2 diabetes are less active and have less physical activity over their lifetime compared with individuals without diabetes [5]. Thus, exercise/physical activity is one of the principal therapies for type 2 diabetes [6]. Exercise modalities, including endurance and resistance training, were employed to improve metabolic control and to ameliorate the progression of DM-related complications [1, 5–7]. Aerobic exercise with low-to-moderate intensity of physical activity (of 40–70% VO_{2max}) done daily in 30-min sessions is strongly recommended [5, 6, 8]. The amount of muscle mass used over the time of activity is beneficial to utilize glycogen in the liver and muscle for improving insulin resistance [9]. However, heavy physical labor and unsafe work environments may more likely lead to musculoskeletal damage [8]. Therefore, it is important to identify a mode of physical activity that can safely and effectively maximize caloric expenditure [10]. Walking is the most commonly performed mode of activity for those with diabetes and is the most convenient low-impact mode of physical activity [6, 7]. However, because of complications or coexisting conditions such as peripheral neuropathy or degenerative arthritis or foot problems, those with type 2 diabetes may need to do nonweight-bearing activities [6]. No matter what exercise mode is chosen, sustaining a lifelong physical activity habit is important [11]. Several risk factors, including glucose levels, blood pressure, lipid/cholesterol profile, and body mass index (BMI), are reportedly improved with these modes of exercise [1, 4, 6, 8, 11]. However, although not all studies demonstrate an improvement in risk factors, they consistently note improvement in complications and a reduction of DM incidence [1]. Therefore, there is convincing evidence that exercise, with or without specific improvements to traditional DM-related risk factors, is an effective therapy for the management of DM [1].

Studies demonstrated that the pathophysiology of type 2 diabetes appears to involve defects in both insulin action (insulin resistance) and secretion (insulin deficiency). The insulin receptor substrate has been postulated to be involved in insulin resistance. Insulin secretion is abnormal in type 2 diabetes patients, with the first phase of insulin release generally being absent [12]. Acute exercise can favorably change abnormal blood glucose and insulin resistance in type 2 diabetes due to its synergistic action with insulin in insulin-sensitive tissues. Furthermore, chronic regular exercise is imperative to sustaining glucose-lowering effects and improving insulin sensitivity while promoting beneficial physiological changes in patients with type 2 diabetes [7, 11]. These include lower resting and submaximal heart rate, increased stroke volume and cardiac output, enhanced oxygen extraction, and lower resting and exercise blood pressure [4, 8, 10, 12].

Parallel to weight-bearing activities such as walking and nonweight-bearing activities such as stationary cycling, swimming, or aquatic activities, Tai Chi exercise is not only a low-impact mode of physical activity with slow and gentle movements [13], but it is also a physical activity that uses muscle mass [14, 15]. Therefore, it could be said that Tai Chi exercise has the qualities of both weight-bearing activities and nonweight-bearing activities. In addition, Tai Chi exercise has effects on the health outcomes of patients with chronic diseases and in particular, benefits patients with cardiac diseases [16]. The other physiological characteristics and beneficial effects of Tai Chi exercise on health are enhanced cardiovascular function, increased strength, increased balance, decreased falls, reduced pain perception, reduced anxiety, and improved self-efficiency [13]. Hence, Tai Chi exercise might be safer and more effective for patients with type 2 diabetes as compared to other exercises.

Despite the evidence that Tai Chi exercise promotes muscle strength in patients with type 2 diabetes [15], the question of whether it could be a therapy for type 2 diabetes has not been studied before. If Tai Chi exercise could decrease blood glucose and especially play an effective role in pathophysiology by improving the insulin resistance of patients with type 2 diabetes, it would be an appropriate exercise mode for patients with type 2 diabetes. Thus, the purpose of the current study was to study the changes in blood glucose of patients with type 2 diabetes through 8 weeks of Tai Chi exercise, and to explain its potential mechanics by analyzing changes in insulin receptor activities which may play a central role as an intermediary step in the muscle glucose transport process [17].

Methods

Subjects

Community-dwelling elders were recruited through questionnaire administration and follow-up interviews after their basic information was obtained from their medical examination records. Subjects were not included in this investigation if they reported any of the following conditions: diabetic neuropathy, fundus hemorrhage, and foot ulceration. After completing a detailed questionnaire on health condition, diet, medical history, lifestyle, and menstrual status, 12 older women, aged 58–75 (66.5 $\pm$ 8.5) years, with BMI 26.1 $\pm$ 2.2, and a history of DM not longer than 2 (1.6 ± 0.4) years, were recruited into the experiment. Five of the subjects had no drug treatments, while the other 7 had oral drug treatments which were not changed during the whole training period. None of them had regular physical exercise before the study.

During the 1st week of experimentation, the subjects had more diet than usual as assessed by self-report. All the participants were instructed not to change their usual dietary habits during the training period.

The participants signed an informed consent. The study was approved by the local institutional review board.

Exercise Protocol

The subjects were trained in Tai Chi exercise lasting for 30 min beginning at about 6:30 every morning during 8 weeks. The exercise was organized and monitored by one qualified Tai Chi instructor. Polar heart rate monitors (Polar Electro, Finland) were used to monitor heart rates so that a 70% maximum heart rate for each subject was maintained for at least 10 min in each exercise. The maximum heart rate was calculated using the formula (220-age) which is widely used in exercise prescription.

A single bout exercise was organized in the morning of the day immediately after the 8-week intervention. In this exercise, the subjects performed the Tai Chi routines twice continuously, lasting for about 12 min, while Polar heart rate monitors were used to ensure that a 70% maximum heart rate for each subject lasted for at least 5 min.

Data Collection

Elbow venous blood samples were collected (4 ml) three times: under empty stomach condition during resting in the morning of the day immediately before (first time) and after (second time) the 8-week Tai Chi intervention, and immediately after the single bout Tai Chi exercise (third time) which was arranged when the third time elbow venous blood samples had been collected. The blood samples were poured into glass test tubes with heparin for anticoagulant. They were then kept refrigerated under low temperature ($-30°C$) until they were measured the day after the acute exercise test. All tests were operated by the Experiment Center of Su-Bei People's Hospital in Yang-Zhou City. The experimental conditions including the place, the laboratory assistants, and the series of instruments used were the same during all the three testing times.

The blood glucose measurement was conducted using the oxidation method with the auto biochemical analysis instrument (7170, Hitachi Limited Corporation).

The insulin was measured using the radioimmunoassay method by ^{125}I-labelled insulin radioimmunoassay kit (Chinese Institute of Atomic Energy, China). The red cell insulin receptor measurement adopted the Gambhir method [18]. Meanwhile, the total blood insulin receptor kit (Chengdu Huaxi Diabetes Research Institute, China) was used in the measurement. Finally, the γ-count instrument (GC-911, Institute of China University of Science and Technology, China Isotope Company, China) was employed as radio counter. The steps in the red cell insulin receptor measurement and computation were performed according to the kit instructions.

Statistics

All variables were presented as means and standard deviations (SD). Changes from the 8-week and acute Tai Chi exercise were analyzed by paired samples t test to detect differences in blood glucose, insulin levels, high- and low-affinity insulin receptor numbers (r_1, r_2), and receptor binding capacity (R_1, R_2) before and after the 8 weeks, and after the single bout exercise. The statistical significance level was set at $p < 0.05$. The statistical program SPSS 10.0 (SPSS, Chicago, Ill., USA) for Windows was used for data evaluation.

Results

The blood glucose measured after the 8-week Tai Chi intervention was significantly lower ($p < 0.05$) than that measured before the intervention. The blood glucose after the single bout Tai Chi exercise increased significantly ($p < 0.05$) as compared to the data measured before the exercise.

The high- and low-affinity insulin receptor numbers (r_1, r_2) and the low-affinity insulin receptor binding capacity (R_2) after the 8-week Tai Chi intervention were found to increase significantly ($p < 0.05$) compared with the data measured before the intervention, indicating that insulin receptor activities were increased and therefore insulin sensitivity was improved. Simultaneously, all the r_1 and r_2 as well as R_1 and R_2 after the single bout exercise increased significantly ($p < 0.05$) compared with the data measured before the exercise, also indicating that there was significant improvement in insulin action.

The serum insulin measured after the 8-week Tai Chi intervention was significantly higher ($p < 0.05$) than that measured before the intervention. However, the single bout Tai Chi exercise did not significantly ($p > 0.05$) increase the serum insulin. The insulin secretion was found to maintain its normal levels (5–20 mU/l) in all three cases.

The BMI of the subjects, which did not decrease ($p > 0.05$), was still higher than the normal value of 25 as classified by WHO during the Geneva Congress of Specialists in 1997 (table 1).

Discussion

The regulation of blood glucose requires a coordinated interaction between several tissues, and this process is mediated by the release of and response to the hormone insulin which in turn triggers an increase in glucose uptake in the target tissues, muscles and fats, as well as the suppression of hepatic glucose release [12]. The relative capacity of insulin to promote a decrease in blood glucose is referred to as insulin sensitivity. The study of insulin sensitivity in humans typically involves the investigation of insulin action in skeletal muscles, which accounts for 75% of glucose disposal. Type 2 diabetes is characterized by skeletal muscle insulin resistance and impaired glucose metabolism [9, 19]. In vivo, muscle insulin sensitivity is regulated on a long-term basis by factors such as

Table 1. Effect of Tai Chi exercise on blood glucose, insulin receptor numbers, and blood insulin in type 2 DM (n = 12)

	Resting before 8 weeks	Resting after 8 weeks	After the single bout exercise
Blood glucose, M	7.75 ± 0.96	6.97 ± 1.06*	7.73 ± 1.15[#]
$R_1 \times 10^{-10}$, M	0.88 ± 0.11	0.92 ± 0.13	2.15 ± 0.18[#]
$R_2 \times 10^{-9}$, M	3.61 ± 0.75	5.87 ± 0.91*	7.53 ± 1.23[#]
r_1, sites	23 ± 8	36 ± 8*	71 ± 11[#]
r_2, sites	803 ± 213	1083 ± 253*	1460 ± 337[#]
Insulin, mU/l	10.03 ± 2.59	11.96 ± 2.01*	11.47 ± 2.29
BMI	26.1 ± 2.2	25.8 ± 2.6	

*p < 0.05 vs. resting before the 8-week training; [#]p < 0.05 vs. resting after the 8-week training.

obesity, and it is altered in a more rapid manner by changes in dietary habits and physical activity [19]. Significant evidence suggests that the acute and chronic regulation of insulin receptor function contributes to alterations in insulin sensitivity and glucose homeostasis. Insulin sensitivity is determined by the number and binding affinity of insulin receptors [20].

Effect of Regular Tai Chi Exercise on Type 2 Diabetes

In the present study, we found that blood glucose was decreased by regular Tai Chi exercise. Further exploration of the alteration of insulin sensitivity revealed that it was significantly increased in association with the increase in the number and binding affinity of insulin receptors, whereas serum insulin was maintained within normal levels as was before the test.

Insulin receptor defect is the risk factor in the pathology of type 2 diabetes [20]. However, the 8-week Tai Chi exercise evidently increased both the numbers and binding capacity of insulin receptors. It demonstrated that regular Tai Chi exercise is good for type 2 diabetics to improve their insulin sensitivities.

It has been reported that controlled obesity could decrease blood glucose in type 2 diabetes [9]. Therefore, exercise was widely perceived to be beneficial for blood glucose control and weight loss in patients with type 2 diabetes. Based on the WHO classification of body mass indexes, all subjects in this test were overweight because their BMIs were above 25. Although the 8-week Tai Chi exercise did not make their BMI decrease evidently, a decreasing trend was found. Studies indicate that long-term (more than 4 months) exercise plays an important role in the treatment of type 2 diabetes and may protect against the development of cardiovascular diseases by improving lipid metabolism [11]. Although the 8-week Tai Chi exercise did not decrease BMI evidently, it demonstrated a decrease in blood glucose. In other words, it indicated that regular Tai Chi exercise could have a steady influence on reducing blood glucose in type 2 diabetes.

Although clinical trials on the effects of exercise in patients with type 2 diabetes have conflicting results as to whether exercise training indeed reduces the risk of diabetic complications, no significant changes in body mass were noted. The possible reasons for this are as follows: (1) the exercise interventions were of relatively short duration and involved only moderate amounts of exercise, and (2) for relatively inactive people, increasing physical activity can result in an increase in lean body mass. Therefore, exercise should be viewed as beneficial on its own and not merely as a tool for weight loss [21]. Finally, promoting insulin sensitivity in the skeletal muscles of type 2 diabetics by Tai Chi exercise [15] might contribute to the improvement of their glucose metabolism [19] through the strengthening of the said muscles.

Effect of Single Bout Tai Chi Exercise on Type 2 Diabetes

Monitoring the intensity of physical activity in persons with type 2 diabetes may require the use of heart rate or ratings of perceived exertion. Activities of moderate intensity (60–80% of maximum heart rate, 50–74% $\dot{V}O_{2max}$) with mild changes in heart rate, blood pressure, and aerobic exercise are usually recommended for type 2 diabetics in order to avoid further coronary artery damage [1, 6, 7].

In our single bout Tai Chi exercise test, a 70% maximum heart rate of each subject has been maintained within 5–6 min for a total of 12 min. This was consistent with the result that the Tai Chi routine practice is a light to moderate intensity exercise [22].

A single bout of exercise acutely improves glucose uptake-specific glucose effectiveness and insulin sensitivity in individuals with normal glucose tolerance in an intensity-dependent manner [23]. Single bout Tai Chi exercise advanced insulin receptor affinity and further improved insulin sensitivity based on significantly increasing the number of insulin receptors and their binding capacity while maintaining the normal serum insulin. Simultaneously, the blood glucose did not decrease, and in fact, it exhibited a slight increase. This result further indicates that the exercise intensity of the Tai Chi routine is enough to stimulate glucose release and utilization, which has a positive effect on blood glucose control according to the increase in insulin sensitivity and decrease in resting blood glucose.

It is generally necessary to increase the safety and efficacy of exercise as both a treatment and a cardiac monitoring strategy for patients with diabetes [8, 10]. Lower-intensity activities afford a more comfortable level of exertion and enhance the likelihood of adherence while lessening the likelihood of musculoskeletal injury and foot trauma [8]. Hence, performing gentler Tai Chi movements which are done in a more relaxed manner should be favorable in controlling heart rates and adjusting the central nervous system to control the blood glucose [24] while enhancing at the same time the regulation of energy balance and peripheral metabolism through the monitoring of insulin sensitivity [25]. The use of many muscles in Tai Chi movements may further enhance blood glucose utilization. Therefore, Tai Chi exercise should be recommended for patients with type 2 diabetes because of its efficacy in controlling blood glucose and, as a gentle mode of exercise, for its safety in avoiding physical injuries.

Conclusion

The 8-week Tai Chi intervention provides evidence of Tai Chi's benefits among older women with type 2 diabetes. Particularly, the 8-week regular Tai Chi exercise decreased blood glucose effectively while maintaining normal insulin levels. Increasing insulin sensitivity might be the primary mechanism which effectively improves the blood glucose metabolism in type 2 diabetes.

References

1   Frier B, Yang Pearl, Taylor AW: Diabetes, aging and physical activity. Eur Rev Aging Phys Act 2006;3:63–73.
2   Correa-Rotter R, González-Michaca L: Early detection and prevention of diabetic nephropathy: A challenge calling for mandatory action for Mexico and the developing world. Kidney Int Suppl 2005;98:S69–S75.
3   Boyle JP, Honeycutt AA, Narayan KM, Hoerger TJ, Geiss LS, Chen H, Thompson TJ: Projection of diabetes burden through 2050: impact of changing demography and disease prevalence in the U.S. Diabetes Care 2001;24:1936–1940.
4   Kernan-Schroeder D, Cunningham M: Glycemic Control and Beyond: The ABCs of Standards of Care for Type 2 Diabetes and Cardiovascular Disease. J Cardiovasc Nurs 2002;16:44–54.
5   Østergård T, Jessen N, Schmitz O, Mandarino LJ: The effect of exercise, training, and inactivity on insulin sensitivity in diabetics and their relatives: what is new? Appl Physiol Nutr Metab 2007;32:541–548.
6   Kirk AF, Barnitt J, Mutrie N: Physical activity consultation for people with Type 2 diabetes. Evidence and guidelines. Diabet Med 2007;24:809–816.
7   Nakhanakhup C, Moungmee P, Appell HJ, Duarte JA: Regular physical exercise in patients with type 2 diabetes mellitus. Eur Rev Aging Phys Act 2006;3:10–19.
8   Hu G, Lakka TA, Kilpelainen TO, Tuomilehto J: Epidemiological studies of exercise in diabetes prevention. Appl Physiol Nutr Metab 2007;32:583–595.
9   Toledo FG, Menshilcova EV, Ritov VB, Azuma IC, Radikova Z, Delany J, Keley DE: Effects of physical activity and weight loss on skeletal muscle mitochondria and relationship with glucose control in type 2 diabetes. Diabetes 2007;56:2142–2147.
10   McDonnell ME: Combination therapy with new targets in Type 2 diabetes: A review of available agents with a focus on pre-exercise adjustment. J Cardiopulm Rehabil Prev 2007;27:193–201.

11 Cauza E, Hanusch-Enserer U, Strasser B, Kostner K, Dunky A, Haber P: The metabolic effects of long term exercise in Type 2 diabetes patients. Wien Med Wochenschr 2006;156:515–519.

12 Reaven GM: Syndrome X. Clin Diabetes 1994;12:32–36.

13 Kuramoto AM: Therapeutic benefits of Tai Chi exercise: research review. WMJ 2006;105:42–46.

14 Qin L, Choy W, Leung K, Leung PC, Au S, Hung W, Dambacher M, Chan K: Beneficial effects of regular Tai Chi exercise on musculoskeletal system. J Bone Miner Metab 2005;23:186–190.

15 Orr R, Tsang T, Lam P, Comino E, Singh MF: Mobility impairment in type 2 diabetes: association with muscle power and effect of Tai Chi intervention. Diabetes Care 2006;29:2120–2122.

16 Cheng TO: Tai Chi: The Chinese ancient wisdom of an ideal exercise for cardiac patients. Int J Cardiol 2007;117:293–295.

17 Juan CC, Chang CL, Chuang TY, Huang SW, Kwok CF, Ho LT: Insulin sensitivity and resistin expression in nitricoxide-deficient rats. Diabetologia 2006;49:3017–3026.

18 Gambhir KK: Insulin radioreceptor assay for human erythrocytes. Clin Chem 1977;2:1590.

19 Corcoran MP, Lemon-fava, Fieding RA: Skeletal muscle lipid deposition and insulin resistance: effect of dietary fatty acids and exercise. Am J Clin Nutr 2007;85:662–677.

20 Youngren JF: Review: Regulation of insulin receptor function. Cell Mol Life Sci 2007;64:873–891.

21 Boulé NG, Haddad E, Kenny GP, Wells GA, Sigal RJ: Effects of exercise on glycemic control and body mass in type 2 diabetes mellitus, A Meta-analysis of Controlled Clinical Trials. JAMA 2001;286:1218–1227.

22 Taylor-Piliae RE, Froelicher ES: Effectiveness of Tai Chi exercise in improving aerobic capacity: a meta-analysis. J Cardiovasc Nurs 2004;19:48–57.

23 Hayashi Y, Nagasaka S, Takahashi N, Kusaka L, Ishibashi S, Numao S, Lee DJ, Taki Y, Ogata H, Tokuyama K, Tanaka K: A single bout of exercise at higher intensity enhances glucose effectiveness in sedentary men. J Clin Endocrinol Metab 2005;90:4035–4040.

24 Motivala SJ, Sollers J, Thayer J, Irwin MR: Tai Chi Chih acutely decreases sympathetic nervous system activity in older adults. J Gerontol A Biol Sci Med Sci 2006;61:1177–1180.

25 Diamant M: Brain insulin signalling in the regulation of energy balance and peripheral metabolism. Ideggyogy Sz 2007;60:97–108.

Jing Hao Wang, PhD
Faculty of Sports Science, South China Normal University
Guangzhou (China)
Tel. +86 020 3931 0271, Fax +86 020 3931 0272, E-Mail tyxbg@scnu.edu.cn

Author Index

Subject Index

Self-regulation, learning 169
Sensory organization test (SOT), balance
    evaluation 116, 118, 119
Sleep stability, heart failure and Tai Chi
    outcomes 199, 203–205
Stepping, *see* Foot movement

Tai Chi (TC)
    guidelines for beginners 67, 68
    overview of benefits 40, 41, 158–160
    styles 12, 13
    traditional curriculum

choreographed form movement 67, 68
    overview 65, 66
    Qigong meditation 66
Tibialis anterior, Tai Chi effects on response
    time 88, 94–99

Vestibular system, balance control and Tai
    Chi 120, 121
Visual system, balance control and Tai Chi
    120
$\dot{V}O_2$, *see* Oxygen uptake

Walking, *see* Foot movement